Book cover design by Cara Finch

Dedication

To our families whose
Love and beauty sustains us,
To our ancestors whose courage and vision
Has shown us the way,
To our progeny
Whose lives dream and arch into the future;
To all the hues and faces of humanity
With whom we share this inner luminosity and journey.

I

II

WHY DARKNESS MATTERS: The Power of Melanin in the Brain
(New and Expanded Edition)

TABLE OF CONTENTS

Edward Bruce Bynum, Ph.D., ABPP, Editor

Table of Figures and Illustrations...v

Preface to the New Edition..............Edward Bruce Bynum, Ph.D.......1

Introduction :The Neuromelanin Hypothesis..................... Edward Bruce Bynum, Ph.D..5

Chapter 1. Neuromelanin: A Highly Sensitized Sensory-Motor Network...T. Owens Moore, Ph.D...17

Chapter 2. Neuromelanin: What Is Its Importance In Neural Tissue ?.......Ann C. Brown, Ph.D..69

Chapter 3. The Clinical Use of Bliss: A Standardized Technique For Conscious Intervention Into The Functions Of The Autonomic Nervous System................Edward Bruce Bynum, Ph.D......................................125

Chapter 4. Neuromelanin : A Black Gate Threshold; I33 Tissue of Heru, Historical, Neurophysiological And Clinical Psychological Issues................................Richard D. King, M.D..178

Postscript ....Edward Bruce Bynum,Ph.D....244

Glossary..250

Brief Autobiographical statements by the authors......................266

Selected Furthur Readings……………………………………………………………..

Brief Autobiographical Statements by the Authors………………………………..

IV

Figures and Illustrations

Chapter 1.
Figure 1. Comparison between the morphology of a skin cell (melanocyte) and brain cell (neuron)

Figure 2. An immunocytochemical technique used to stain for tyrosine hydroxylase in the substantia nigra.

Chapter 2.
Figure 1. Cast of the ventricles of the brain (lateral view)

Figure 2. Cast of the ventricles of the brain (dorsal view)

Chapter 3.
Chart I. Schemata of human nervous system

Chart II. Partial list of stress modulated diseases and symptoms
Graph 1. Sagittal section of human brain with twelve cell neuromelanin foci

Graph 2. Limbic system primary structures

Chart III. Human brain stem with twelve areas of high concentrations of pigmented cells
Graph 3. The twelve neuromelanin foci identified

Chapter 4.
Figure 1. Representation of Anu

Figure 2. The Spirit of the Sun

Figure 3. Triune god of the Osirian Resurrection

Figure 4. Osiris Khenti Amentt

Figure 5. Upper Register-First Group of Divinities

Preface to the New Edition

"The mothering earth is dark,
And, deep inside me, I am dark".
 -Pablo Neruda, 'I ask for silence'
 Extravagaria

It has been nearly a decade since the first edition of **WHY DARKNESS MATTERS:The Power of Melanin in the Brain** came to the attention of the general public. The book was designed to introduce the public to the science behind the subject of melanin and neuromelanin free of the political and ideological concerns that had surrounded much of its presentation in the American media. In particular the role of melanin and neuromelanin in neurology, neuroanatomy, medicine, embryology, evolution and philosophy itself was a central goal of the book.

In its four chapters the authors, who represented perspectives in clinical psychology, psychiatry, neuroscience and neuroanatomy, each sought to bring forward relevant well documented information to a sometimes controversial and misunderstood field. Each spoke a little to the clinical and political impact of surface melanin but placed more emphasis on the deeper implications of melanin and neuromelanin in the functions of embryology, medicine and neuroscience.

While acknowledging the role that variable surface or skin melanin has in political and social discourse, this surface melanin was differentiated from brain or neuromelanin. We stressed how neuromelanin increases in density and amount as we ascend the evolutionary ladder from the simple vertebrates through the mammalian lines up to the primates and culminating in man. We brought attention to the fact that melanin converts energy from one state to another, e.g. thermal to vibration to sound etc. We emphasized how melanin, from both our own and a scientific perspective, was not merely a "waste product" but appears to serve complex protective functions in certain circumstances.

Research has continued in this area from that first edition with contributions occurring on a world wide stage confirming the complexity and range of this biopolymer in the human brain. Much of this research has focused on the role of melanin and neuromelanin especially in neurodegenerative disorders such as Parkinson's disease (Zecca et al, 2006; Fedorow et al, 2005). It was one of the authors here, Dr. Ann Brown, an anatomist/hematologist, who also suggested that given their symptomatic manifestations that there appears to be a clinical relationship between neuromelanin, Parkinson's and Alzheimer's disease. Others have gone in different directions and explored neuromelanin's melanic structure (Engelen et al;2012), its biosynthetic pathway(Wakamatsu et al; 2012) and its immune system implications(Oberlander, et al; 2011).

There have seen a series on melanin conferences in the United States that have sought to bring the findings of this scientific area to the interested public as well as international professional scientific conferences for researchers in this widening field, e.g., International Conference on Pigment Development workshops, as well as a research oriented journal, *Pigment Cell & Melanoma Research*. Many of these are medically oriented and will have even more relevance in the future as climate change affects our planet and more people are exposed to the sun's ultraviolent radiation effects on the skin.

New published work by some of the authors has continued the line of inquiry on the apparent semi-conductive and subtle bioluminous characterists of neuromelanin that appear to have been observed in the contemplative disciplines and traditions and so taken the study in more modern directions , e.g., **DARK LIGHT CONSCIOUSNESS; Melanin, Serpent Power, and the Luminous Matrix of Reality** (Bynum, 2012).

The wider implications of neuromelanin, its demonstrated photo-active and semi-conductive properties and also certain currents within the perennial philosophy had been briefly brought to the fore in the first edition, especially by Dr. Richard D. King. Given that melanin and neuromelanin is "black" partially means that it absorbs light or photons and converts it to other energy states (Barr, 1983), identifying it as a form of energy conductivity and bioluminosity that surely interacts with consciousness. We asked how does consciousness interact with or is implicated in the neurodynamics of neuromelanin and neurogenesis or the growth of new neural cells. We wondered how the "inner" warm dark matter of neuromelanin was related in any way to the "outer" 'cold dark matter' of the cosmos. Essentially how is it that a dark information processing brain is interpreting a dark and perhaps in some way conscious cosmos.

Certain questions were raised but certainly not answered in the book such as exactly what *is* consciousness and how is the bioluminosity of neuromelanin related to the "*inner light*" perceived and made reference to in innumerable psychospiritual traditions and experiences across the world. We do sense that in some way this dark living innermost aspect of us is resonate with the vast dark matter that seems to compose the external universe. 'As above, so below; as within, so without' is a confession and principal of the ancient Hermetic corpus, as is the maximum that ultimately 'All is Mind'. This was the revelation of the primogenitor Tehuti on the banks of the Nile by the pyramids over 5000 years ago that set the stage and has guided humankind on its present course of scientific and philosophical thought.

The Vedantic solution to the apparent difference between matter and consciousness is an elegant one. That is to say that matter itself appears to be a form of veiled consciousness. In contemporary physics it is already implicit that there is a subtle 'observer' embedded in Relativity theory and numerous schools in quantum mechanics tacitly admit that consciousness is entangled with the observations and behavior of the minutest forms of energetic particles.

With this edition of **WHY DARKNESS MATTERS: The Power of Melanin in the Brain** we have greatly expanded the glossary and added an extended list of selected readings related to this broad subject. The study will go through many other future changes and expansions as it is further integrated into science and medicine. This is to be expected and a welcome sign of a maturing field. Despite its lineage in the form of an ancient scientific and philosophical study of darkness and light that interfaces with human life and consciousness, it is still in many ways only in its infancy.

References

Barr, F.E., 1983. Melanin: The organizing molecule. Medical Hypotheses 11: 1-140.

Bynum, E.B., 2012. **DARK LIGHT CONSCIOUSNESS: Melanin, Serpent Power and the Luminous Matrix of Reality**. Inner Traditions & bear company, Rochester, VT.

Engelen, M., Bellei,C., Vanna,R. et al 2012. "Neuromelanins of human brain have soluble and insoluble components with dolichols attached to the melanic structure". Plos One 7(11):e48490, doi:10. 1371/journal.pone 0048490, Nov 5.

Fedorow, H.,Tribl, F., Halliday, G., Gerlach, M., Reiderer, P., Double,K. L. 2005. :Neuromelanin in human dopamine neurons: comparison with peripheral melanins and relevance to Parkinson's". Progress in Neurobiology, Feb: 75(2), 109-24.

Oberlander,U., et al 2011. "Neuromelanin is an immune stimulator for dendritic cells in vitro". BMC Neuroscience12:116.

Wakamatsu, K., Murase,T. ,Zucca, F.,Zecca, L., Shosuke, I. 2012. "Biosynthetic pathway to neuromelanin and its aging process", in Pigment Cell & Melanoma Research, Vol. 25, Issue 6, 792-803. John Wiley & Sons: Hoboken, NJ.

INTRODUCTION

The Neuromelanin Hypothesis

"All traces of psychological subjects including 'psychotherapy' were practiced in Africa by the Egyptians and long pre-dated the Greek, Roman, and Hebrew tradition in which much modern western psychology is rooted. Imhotep...(is) the first figure of a physician to stand out clearly from the midst of antiquity."
        A.K. Tay, Psychology in Africa, The Unesco Courier

The thrust of this book **WHY DARKNESS MATTERS** on the reality of melanin in the brain or the neuromelanin hypothesis is to acquaint a larger audience with the history, complexity and importance of this vital and at times controversial area of science, psychology and neuroscience. A searching review of its contents however will quickly reveal that it touches upon a number of sensitive areas in the living fabric of our society and by historical extension the dynamics of many other contemporary cultures and sociopolitical worlds. The importance of variable surface skin melanin in Western and European influenced societies and the subsequent psychodynamics of racism and color are well known and documented (Akbar, 1984; Fanon, 1967;Welsing, 1991). Indeed this aspect of the phenomenon has been the source of not only almost endless academic debates but also volatile political and social movements. Anyone who is only vaguely aware of the confluence of race and ethnic realities in the United States alone cannot fail to see its impact and current expressions. Its dynamics were deeply woven into the intimate social and economic fabric of the republic from the earliest days of its existence (Bennett, 1966; Stampp, 1956). We are almost fixated on this and its cyclical eruption in the streets, classrooms and courts of America. We have had great difficulty seeing beyond it. The attempts to become a "color blind" society, while noble in impulse, have only painfully avoided certain issues, made others worse, and by fixation on mere surface skin dynamics, made us blind to other, perhaps deeper more luminous realities. This volume will go in an altogether different direction and offer a new paradigm from which to observe and experience this phenomenon.

The seminal influence of inner melanin or brain melanin in human consciousness is not as well known as surface skin melanin and yet implicates all human beings without regard to so call "race" or ethnic diversity. This new wave of academic and clinical interest in melanin is actually the second wave, the first occurring in the 1980's. Each wave takes us further and deeper into the ocean of this area of science. The first wave sometimes hit upon the reefs of political polemics due to certain exaggerated claims made for it and at times the lack of clear scientific and clinical depth in its presentation to the public. It was a risky and controversial area to study given the climate at that time, a climate that persists to some degree even today. However it must also be emphasized here that certain problems arose in its study because of **the independent conceptual vision it unfolded for African peoples with the enormous potential and implications it has for science and society**. You see it was not so much the "objective" data that was in question but rather the psychohistoricly informed scientific lens through which the data was focused that was crucial. It suggested neither a psychodynamic nor cognitive behavioral view of mind and consciousness, but rather a scientific vision that was not tacitly even within the sphere of Eurocentric intellectual thought. It harkened back to older, more expansive paradigms of mind, life and science that illuminated and held sway over the ancient world for millennia. It also opened a pathway out of the obsessive preoccupation with the painful but addictively familiar framing of issues of race and color around which many individuals and even institutions were and are focused. These powerful interests made for a difficult launch in a new direction. Hopefully this new wave can steer clear of these reefs and stay true to the potential it carries for both science and African American studies in particular. This volume makes its contribution in the area of neuroscience.

Neuroscience was actually born from the womb of Kemetic Egyptian neuroanatomy. By the 18th dynasty there were thousands of medical papyri used in the medical "houses of life' or per ankh which became the model for later Greek medical practice (Ghalioungui, 1973; Breasted, 1984). Indeed due to the necessity for both battle field trauma medicine and the elaborate process of mummification a great deal was known about human anatomy (Finch, 1990). Sadly enough of the thousands of medical texts written only 10 have come down to us, of which the Edwin Smith and
"Ebbers papyrus are the most well known. The Edwin Smith "medical" papyrus is actually a surgical treatise and a copy of a much older papyrus dating back centuries and covers only the head and neck. The other parts of the text unfortunately are lost to history. It details some 50 specific anatomical sites in the face, neck and cranium alone. The Kemetic Egyptians were well aware of the cerebral gyruses and the meninges of the brain, the dura mater, pia mater, and arachnoid along with certain injury related behavioral expressions in clinical practice. They were also aware of the crucial importance of the cerebrospinal fluid that bathes the brain, the inner mid-brain regions and the spinal cord (Finch, 1990). Kemetic medical anatomy identified well over 200 clinical sites of which almost 100 are located in this surviving text. Even after the geopolitical and military fall of

Kemet it remained the graduate school of the ancient western world for the Greeks and Romans. As Homer said in the Odyssey," In medical knowledge, Egypt leaves the rest of the world behind". It was not until the 19th century that the amount and detail of such medical knowledge was surpassed in Europe. In this sense neuroscience has been a living part of medicine and psychology from the earliest eras of African civilization and underlies much of contemporary medical practice.

Traditionally Western science has adopted two divergent stances in regard to these two branches of African medical and psychological science. Either it has completely ignored it despite its existence as evidenced in the above data on the African background in medical science in both internal medicine and the fundementals of neuroscience, both of which are rarely if ever mentioned in our standard medical and scientific texts. Indeed the fact that the unconscious was actually discovered in ancient Egypt and given the names of the Primeveal Waters of Nun and the Amenta (Hourning,1986; King,1990);that Carl Jung's concept of the archetype derives from the north African scholar Saint Augustine's Principales as well as his deriving the notions of anima and animus from the anthropologist Sir Edward Tylor's "study" of Africans in his Primitive Culture(1871); or that the Greek word "psyche" itself is a derivation of the older Egyptian words "Khe" for soul and "Su" for she, Su-Khe(Massey,1881),is an expression of this tendency.Indeed it is either ignored or else the knowledge is greatly distorted and held up to ridicule as simply "primitive" supersition or the "dark sciences" when it comes to the areas of spiritual practice and certain anomalous experiences. Popular movies and other practicing black magic" which the West is both amused by and cultural motifs have a rich history of showing Africans secretely terrified of for many reasons that go beyond the present scope of this book.

The chapters here are organized around the subject of brain melanin or neuromelanin, putting the material in a new light. Melanin as a social and skin perception experience is a complex social, political and cultural phenomenon. Brain or neuromelanin however is an all-together different phenomenon that has less to do with various human prejudices and fears and more to do with human nervous system functioning, evolutionary unfoldment and ultimately, as we shall suggest, consciousness itself. These chapters will unfold sequentially and present in both academic and medical-clinical clarity that melanin and especially neuromelanin, with its affinity for conductivity and luminosity, is present in significant amounts in crucial areas of cerebral and central nervous system functioning in ALL human beings. This has medical, psychological and even spiritual implications.

But what does this mean? Why is it that melanin appears to be an "organizing molecule" in the early embryological and structural unfoldment of higher-level mammalian and primate developmental processes (Barr, 1983)? Is this just a biological artifact or does it imply something deeper about human experience and the process of evolution itself? What does this warm living dark matter have to do, if anything at all, with the ubiquitous cold dark matter of the cosmos? Historically African epistemological paradigms have stressed that the macrocosm reflects the microcosm, that through the principle of correspondence, " as above, so below", "as within, so without". This is the great organizing vision of the primogenitor Tehuti or Thoth who the Greeks would later adopt and call Hermes Mercurius Trismegistus (Chandler, 1999; Copenhaver, 1992; Kybalion, 1940). In contemporary scientific language we would refer to certain aspects of this vision in neuroscience and quantum mechanics as the holonomic paradigm. (Pribram,1991 ; Bohm, 1980).

About the brain itself only a small shore of an almost infinite ocean is presently known. We know that the adult human brain weighs roughly three pounds, has a thick jelly-like consistency and is about ninety percent the content of seawater. It's surface looks somewhat like the bark of a tree from which it derives its Latin name "cortex". It is has two hemispheres and four distinct regions or lobes, the frontal, the occipital, the parietal and the temporal. Each lobe or region has more localized functions and all work in intimate biochemical, bioelectric and resonate coordination with each other. The cortex is that part of the brain that is most developed in modern humans since our ancestors had more primitive aspects of this in their own makeup. This cortex is a folded sheet of neurons with 99% of its thickness between 1 and 4.5 mm. The average thickness is about 2.5mm with regional variations. Thickness is associated with increased "activity". Cortical thinning on the other hand is due generally to disease and/or aging and often specific to regions of the brain rather than global.

The brain is a very versatile and adaptive organ with many redundant features. Research in the neurosciences is always producing fascinating supprises for both the scientist and the general public. Brain imaging devices such as the MRI have revealed that indeed the brains of men and women are different. Men's brains are on average 10% larger than women's while women generally demonstrate more functional connections between the two hemispheres of the brain at the connecting region of the corpus callosum. In certain regions of the brain women show a greater density of neurons and use more areas when solving a problem. Men on the other hand tend to be more focused in specific regions of the brain when working on a cognitive problem. NONE of this implies any inate or ultimate superiority or inferiority between men and women, only diversity and difference related to specific tasks, situations and conditions. There is even evidence indicating that learning new skills actually **increases neuromelanin concentration** in certain regions of this marvelous organ and fountainhead of human intelligence and creativity. This last is a most intriguing finding.

You see despite being hidden from the sun this cortex is dark or "gray" in color because it is rich in neuromelanin or brain melanin and the darker and richer this neuromelanin has become in evolution the more cognitively sophisticated our species has become. Beneath and enfolded within the cortex are the various midbrain limbic structures responsible for modulating our emotional and mammalian experiences. Beneath this is the diencephalon which modulates and regulates sleep, appetite and other sensory and homeostatic functions. The very lowest region includes the reptilian brain. Here the functions of breathing, movement, blood flow, somatic temperature and other primal functions are regulated. Neurons or brain cells with dendrites and axons interconnect and interpenetrate this vast living web of information and energy and radiates the mystery of consciousness. Neuromelanin is an intimate aspect of this bioluminous information process because of its unique biochemical and bioelectrical properties. Needless to say this information process not only interconnects the brain within itself and with the body's other organ systems but also with the wider social, cultural, political, and even solar environment. Each author will explore this phenomenon in a unique way, including its scientific, metapsychological and bioluminious implications.

There will be four chapters that progressively unfold this subject. The chapters all build upon and draw from each other seeking in their integration a paradigm shift in this area because of its importance to all of us both medically and neurologically. Future experimental and observational data will deepen this understanding. There is not enough room in the present volume to address the human body's internal organ systems and the role of melanin in health care. Suffice it to say that melanin is present and plays a significant role in the body's internal organ systems, including the heart, liver, gastrointestinal tract, eyes, skin, sexual organs, and the diffuse neuroendocrine system. This edition will focus primarily on neuroscience and the psychological-psychiatric aspects of this vast discipline.

In particular the chapters will stress that melanin and especially brain or neuromelanin is present in ALL human beings internally as well as externally as a matter of complex biology. It will also be noted that melanin and neuromelanin appear, in crucial ways, to guide human embryological development in the womb and the differentiation of the organ systems (Barr, 1983). Because this process of melanin and neuromelanin is ubiquitous in the higher life forms and that the "higher" the level of nervous system development among all animals, on through the primate family, the higher the amount of neuromelanin in the cerebral structures, it suggests a unique contribution of this paradoxically "dark" but "light" absorbing substance in evolutionary unfoldment. This strongly implies that, contrary to past clinical and academic opinion, neuromelanin is not simply a " waste product" of the system but instead represents a crucial albeit not fully understood process in this complex situation.

At times attention will be focused on the fact that the molecular structure of melanin and neuromelanin demononstrates semi-conductor properties and indeed may be a biological superconductor under certain conditions. In other words it has the capacity for luminosity in restricted settings. Given the affinity of human consciousness for light itself this opens the door to processes that, while rooted in neuroscience, have implications for human consciousness that greatly transcend our current scientific conceptual paradigms and reach into the contemplative traditions and disciplines studied by students of meditation for untold millennia. Melanin is found in the inner workings of our bodies, our organ systems, and our intimate cerebral structures, as well as in the wider solar and cosmic ambience around us. Is there an interface? Is there a connection relevant to human health and psychology?

Professor Tim O. Moore opens with a chapter grounding us in the neural mechanisms underlying these pigmented neurons of the nervous system. Thereafter follows a crucial elaboration of the developmental origins of these neuromelanin neurons and their subsequent distribution throughout the unfolding process of embryogenesis or development in the womb. The role of neuromelanin in sensory and motor functioning and enhancement is presented in this context. From this perspective the neurodegenerative processes found in both Parkinson's and Alzheimers disease are thrown into a new light. The semiconductor and energy transfer properties of neuromelanin are critical in all of these processes. This work represents a continuation of Dr. Moore's earlier work in the **Science of Melanin** (Moore, 1995; 2002).

Professor Ann C. Brown picks up the story by acknowledging that these pigmented organic biopolymers are found not only in the brain, but also in the biosphere, atmosphere, lithosphere and the cosmos itself. Brain melanin is found in crucial areas in the very center of the brain's deep cavities, the mid brain's circumventricular organs. Dr. Brown points out that these sub cortical pigmented nuclei and their "neuron circuitry" are very responsive to the complex plasticity of the cerebral processes and are also implicated in the actual generation of new nerve cells called neurogenesis. Other brain centers are then explored in this clinical and neuroanatomical context that, like in the opening chapter by Professor Moore, extends and reframes our understanding of Parkinson's and Alzheimers disease. African Blacks and Asians have the lowest prevalence of Parkinson's whereas Europeans have the highest levels. What, if any, is the connection here? The influence of diet and nutrician is shown to be crucial in the neurodynamics of neuromelanin.

In a primarily clinical article focused on psychosomatic medicine Edward Bruce Bynum presents a way for the practicing clinician to intervene in the functions of the emotionally reactive autonomic nervous system to affect anxiety mediated somatic and behavioral symptoms. The neural and somatic organ system operations are thought to be deeply influenced by these neuromelanin implicated processes. The role of neuromelanin's semiconductor and bioluminious properties is pivotal. Thereafter follows an elaboration of this perspective from both a present day clinical perspective focusing on the human "emotional brain" or mid brain limbic system and also its connection with other healing and contemplative traditions from diverse peoples of the earth. Many of these ideas were outlined in Dr. Bynum's research on **The African Unconscious** (Bynum, 1999). The bioluminious properties of neuromelanin are seen to modulate our connection to the wider biological and solar ecology. The interwoven fabric of spacetime itself is implicated in this process.

Finally in a clinical and theoretical article drawn from the methodology of dynamic psychiatry Richard D. King explores the historical roots and range of melanin studies from both modern and ancient perspectives. Melanin studies in some form he contends have been part of the medical and sacred study of mankind for millennia, an idea explored in depth in his seminal work **The African Origin of Biological Psychiatry** (King, 1990; 1994). This is what Dr.King terms the Amenta nerve tract of neuromelanin reflected in brain or neural structures and paralleled in the spinal column. His focus is on the first scientific elucidation of this knowledge in the texts and practices of ancient Kemet. Again the macrocosm-microcosm correspondence in the epistemological paradigm of the ancients is seen to be more than relevant to our present day exploration. How inner brain structures reflect outer physical structures in specific ways is the thrust here," as above, so below; as within, so without", a kind of neurocosmology (Siler, 1990). He also concludes that evolution is still active and on going and, like professor Ann Brown, that neurogenesis or new brain cells develop partially under the aegis of this neuromelanin mediated process.

These chapters in combination present a view of this ancient but vast and reemerging field that has implications for many areas of research. This knowledge of the intimate psychoenergetic functioning of neuromelanin in evolution and the neural structures opens the doorway again to cognitive and contemplative disciplines discovered in the early Nile valley civilizations of Kemet that later flowered in the Indus valley of India and the eventually throughout the earth. That rediscovery and its bioluminious potential rooted in the neural network and organ systems of the human body is part of the gift this area of science offers to humanity. Each author is mining a small part of this rich motherload of knowledge and experience for science and perhaps the arts and more. The health of African and African American populations throughout the world is in serious need of both clinical expertise and resources but also a bold new conceptual reorganization that takes into account not only the latest in medical and experimental research, but also the sustained genius of our forbearers who studied the deeper mysteries of the heart and the broader sciences of the mind. It is to that living tradition that this volume is dedicated.

REFERENCES

Akbar,N.,1984 Chains And Images Of Psychological Slavery. Jersey City, NJ: New Mind Productions.

Barr, F.E. 1983 Melanin: The organizing molecule, In D.F. Horrobin (Ed.) Medical Hypotheses, vol. 11, Edinburgh: Chruchill Livingstone, 1-140.

Bennett, L., 1962 Before The Mayflower: A History of the Negro in America. Chicago, Ill.: Johnson Publishing Co.

Breasted , J.H.,1984,The Edwin Smith Papyrus, Birmingham,U.K.; The Classics Medical Library.

Bohm, D 1980 Wholeness and the Implicate Order. London: Routledge & Kegan Paul.

Bynum, E.B. 1999 The African Unconscious: Roots of Ancient Mysticism and Modern Psychology, NYC: Columbia University Teachers College Press.

Chandler, W.B. 1999 Ancient Future: The Teachings and Prophetic Wisdom of the Seven Hermetic Laws of Ancient Egypt, Baltimore, MD; Black Classic Press.

Copenhaver, B.P. Hermetica, London: Cambridge University Press.

Fanon, F.1967 Black Skin, White Masks New York, N.Y.: Grove Press.

Finch, C.S. 1990 The African Background to Medical Science, London, U.K.: Karnak House.

Ghalioungui, P., 1973 The House of Life: Magic and Medical Science in Ancient Egypt, Amsterdam, B.M.: Israel, p.31.

Hourning, E. 1986 The discovery of the unconscious in ancient Egypt. Spring Publication: An annual of Archetypal Psychology and Jungian thought, 16-28.

King, R.D., 1990 The African Origin of Biological Psychiatry, Germantown, TN: Seymour Smith.

King, R.D. 1994 Melanin: A Key to Freedom, Hampton, VA: U.B. & U.S. Communications Systems, Inc. Publishers.

Kybalion, 1940 Hermetic Philosophy, Chicago, Ill: Masonic Publication Society.

Massey, G. 1881 The Book of Beginnings (vols 1,2)London: Williams and Norgate.

Moore, T.O. 1995The Science of Melanin: Dispelling the Myths, Silver Spring, MD: Becham House Publishers.

Moore, T.O. 2002 Dark Matters, Dark Secrets, Redman, GA: Zaman Press.

Pribram, K.H. 1991 Brain and Perception: Holonomy and Structure in Figural Processing. Hillsdale, NJ: Erlbaum.

Siler, T. 1990 Breaking the mind Barrier: The Artscience of Neurocosmology, NYC: Touchstone Books/Simon & Schuster.

Stampp, K.M., 1956 The Peculiar Institution: Slavery in the Ante-Bellum South. New York, N.Y.: Vintage Books.

Tylor, E. B., 1871 Primitive Culture. Cited in J.S. Mbiti (1969) African Religions and Philosophy.Portsmouth, NH: Heinemann.

Welsing, F.C. 1991 The Isis Papers: The Keys to the Colors, Chicago, Ill: Third World Press.

WHY DARKNESS MATTERS: The Power of Melanin in the Brain

"All truth passes through three stages...
First it is ridiculed.
Second it is violently opposed.
Third it is accepted as being self-evident."
           -Arthur Schopenhauer, 1788-1860

"All knowledge is a continuation, acted upon by numerous scholars in the quest
for some portion of the truth. Although we might assume that there are many versions
of an event, in reality they are extenuations and attenuations of the same knowledge."
           -Molefi Kete Asante, <u>Kemet, Afrocenriticity and Knowledge</u>

"From an African-centered perspective, we understand truth to be inseparable
from the search for meaning and purpose –the unique concern of human consciousness. As African scholars, it is our responsibility to create systematic theoretical formulations
which will reveal the truths that enable us to liberate and utilize the energies of our people. In this view, the self-determinist, the revolutionary, and the scholar are one, having the same objective, involved in the same truth-process. The claim that we make is not to spurious "objectivity", but to honesty.

- Marimba Ani, <u>Yurugu: An African-Centered Critique of European Thought and Behavior</u>

CHAPTER 1

Neuromelanin: A Highly Sensitized Sensory-Motor Network
T. Owens Moore, Ph.D.

OVERVIEW
This chapter will explore the neural mechanisms underlying pigmented neurons in the nervous system. In general, the dark pigment deep within the brain (i.e., neuromelanin) has a critical role in promoting an optimal level of nervous system functioning. In this chapter, the developmental origin of neuromelanin, its subsequent distribution within the nervous system, and its biosynthesis within the brain will be reviewed. Experimental research on the biophysical properties of melanin has provided significant information on the supportive role of neuromelanin in the nervous system. Although early research suggested that neuromelanin was a waste product, there is a plethora of recent evidence to dispute this claim. Current research on the biophysical properties of melanin can elucidate the mechanisms by which neuromelanin functions in the nervous system. For example, neuromelanin is an antioxidant that can prevent

cellular damage, it can act as a semiconductor by increasing the speed of nerve impulses, and it can function as an electrochemical transducer to transform physical stimuli into neural activity. The electrochemical transducing capability and the overall biophysical properties of neuromelanin appears to be associated with advanced neural processing in mammals and primates. In sum, this dark matter in the brain is a highly sensitized sensory-motor network.

INTRODUCTION

Melanin is the general term used to describe pigment in humans. In humans, pigments come in various colors that are found inside as well as outside of the human body. This topic has been presented by scholars in numerous fields of study to provide a unique perspective of melanin functioning in humans. For example, chemistry, biology, physics, psychology and neuroscience are areas of study that have contributed to our understanding of the role and significance of melanin in the nervous system (i.e., neuromelanin). An extensive review of the science of melanin has been documented by this author (Moore, 1995; 2002) to validate the numerous roles for melanin in human physiology. The literature reviewed in this chapter will be from experimental animal research and research on neuromelanin in the human nervous system. The reader will gain an understanding on the significance of the dark pigment deep within the brain of humans. The origin, location, biosynthesis and advantages of neuromelanin functioning will be explored.

A MYSTERY UNVEILED

Melanin is a mystery because it is a pigment associated with blackness. In this race conscious society, issues related to Ablackness@ can be a lightening rod for controversy. On one hand, the area of melanin research has been neglected because of the politics of scientific research. Since much of the experimental research has been conducted by non-black scientists, it is this author=s opinion that an objective perspective of this area of research has been neglected. On the other hand, if African-centered scientists explore the area of melanin research with provocative intellectual questions, then they may be labeled as reverse racists or pseudoscientists (de Montellano, 1993) for raising issues that are difficult for non-black scientists to comprehend. The mystery of melanin functioning has been revealed and we can no longer view it as a Awaste product@ in the nervous system (Graham, 1979).

In 1975, Clark, McGee, Nobles and Weems wrote a classic article and presented a very clear and concise analysis of melanin in the central nervous system (CNS). It is known that our CNS performs a critical information processing role which is essential for optimal neurological and metabolic functioning. According to Clark et al., there is a high, positive correlation between specific levels of sensory activity and states of pigmentation that has been examined by neurophysiological, neurochemical and neurohumoral data. These authors were led to believe that melanin refines the CNS and, in so doing, produces a highly sensitized sensory-motor network.

According to Clark et al., the original race was African, and people of African descent exhibit the largest quantity of melanin. The authors make a connection between melanin and CNS functioning by stating that a major portion of the empirical research conducted in African Psychology involves a systematic examination of the relationship between melanocytes and the nerve cells of the CNS. As we will discuss in the next section, both are embryologically-derived from a single neuroblast in the neural crest of the developing human fetus.

ORIGIN OF NEUROMELANIN

Cells in the skin that produce, synthesize and secrete melanin are called melanocytes. Melanocytes, which are found in the basal cell layer and between cells of the epidermis, have dynamic functions because they can change as a result of direct physical stimulation or from the normal aging process. In contrast, pigmented neurons in the nervous system are not commonly named melanocytes because they are less dynamic and more static. Neuromelanin is found in the cytoplasm of pigmented neurons (Bazelon, Fenichel and Randall, 1967), and the presence of neuromelanin is less subject to change.

The amount of neuromelanin in the nervous system is determined by genetics. It is quite clear that the amount of external melanin varies between ethnic groups; however, it is considerably more difficult to measure ethnic variations in the stable nature of internal melanin. Although the term static or stable is used here, it is not implied that neuromelanin levels can never change in an individual. For example, deterioration of neuromelanin-containing brain cells can be caused by drugs, chemicals or the normal aging process. The primary role for melanin in the skin is to protect against ultraviolet radiation. Assuming that ultraviolet radiation does not penetrate the brain, neuromelanin in the nervous system and melanin in the skin have slightly different functional roles. In contrast, an analysis of the origin of internal and external melanin can demonstrate the commonality between the two forms of melanin.

<u>Developmental Embryology</u>

During fertilization, a zygote forms and it divides into three distinct germ layers: the endoderm; the mesoderm; and the ectoderm. To understand the important role of melanin during the early stages of embryonic development, we are interested in the derivatives of the outer embryonic layer - the ectoderm. The ectoderm is composed of three regions: the prospective neural tube; the prospective neural crest; and the prospective epidermis. It is within these three regions that melanin plays its first key role in maintaining life. In the midst of this embryological darkness, an explosion (Big Bang) will occur that will transform the tiny mass of cells into a complex human being.

Each region of the ectoderm is further differentiated into specialized body parts. The *neural tube* is differentiated into the following parts: a) the brain; b) the posterior pituitary gland; c) the optic vesicles; d) the spinal cord; and e) the motor nerves that originate in the ventral portion of the neural tube and innervate muscles. The *neural crest* derivatives consist of cells that migrate to distant parts of the body. These migrating cells form sensory nerves and ganglia, which receive impulses from the following sites: a) sense organs; b) autonomic ganglia; c) the adrenal medulla; d) all of the pigmented retinal cells, which are derived from the neural tube; e) the cartilages in the voice box and head; and f) some of the ectodermal muscles. The *epidermal layer* can be divided into cells derived from epidermal thickenings and those derived from the rest of the epidermis. The thick epidermal derivatives include some of the cranial nerves, the lens of the eye, the olfactory structures, the inner ear, and the taste buds. The remainder of the epidermis forms the following structures: a) the outer layer of the skin; b) the hair and nails; c) the linings of the mouth and anus; and d) the anterior pituitary gland (Oppenheimer and Lefevre, 1984).

Melanin is in numerous locations in the body, and the importance of neuromelanin in brain tissue will be discussed in detail by Brown in Chapter 2. For this section, the reader should be aware of neuromelanin's role during embryogenesis.

<u>Neuromelanin and Embryogenesis</u>

Melanin and neuromelanin are part of the sensory-motor network from the earliest stages of embryogenesis. As mentioned in the previous section, the brain and the spinal cord are formed from the neural tube, the sensory-motor network extends from the neural crest and melanocytes in the skin come from the epidermal layer. Each site is dependent on the presence of melanin for proper physiological functioning.

Since our sensory apparatus is so vital to learning, it begins to develop *in utero* within a couple of months after conception (Hannaford, 1995). Nerves appear three weeks after the egg is fertilized and immediately begin to link up with other nerves. Before birth, we learn about gravity through our vestibular system, and our body becomes a fine tuned sensory receptor for collecting information. During embryogenesis, our sensory-motor system shapes our experience, and we are shaped by the events that occur *in utero*.

The human embryo develops out of a womb of darkness and there is no sunlight available to stimulate the production of melanin inside the fetus or on the external surface of the fetus. All sources of melanin migrate to their destination sites by chemical factors such as neurotrophins (Reichardt and Farinas, 1999). Neurotrophins expressed in targets can promote survival of neurons whose cell bodies are distant ganglia.

Experimental research has shown that extirpation and explanation of the neural crest have revealed that it is the sole source of all pigment cells of the body, except those which differentiate in the retina and are therefore derived from the optic cup (LeDouarin and Kalcheim, 1999). If portions of neural crest cells are removed, body parts would be missing and pigmentation would be absent. On the other hand, grafting tissue from the neural crest onto the embryo can increase pigmented cells.

In sum, the aggregation of heavily melanized cells forms the grossly visible black pigmentation in the developing embryo. Melanin and neurotrophic factors move into the folds of the neural groove and appear to bring the folds of the neural tube together to form the brain and the spinal cord. The formation of the neural crest helps to fuse the neural folds and the nervous system begins to take form and shape.

Sensory Enhancement

The nervous system is divided into the CNS and the peripheral nervous system (PNS). The brain and spinal cord are the main components of the CNS, and the PNS is further divided into the autonomic and the somatic nervous system. The processing of sensory information occurs at every aspect of the nervous system, and the presence of melanin can influence both the development of the nervous system as well as how brain cells integrate sensory information with other physiological systems. For example, the migration of cells to make the melanocytes in the skin shed light on the connection between the skin as an extension of the nervous system. Melanocytes are multidendritic cells derived from the neural crest that look very similar to the structure of nerve cells in the brain. Fig. 1 illustrates a comparison of the two cell types. Neurons in the brain and melanocytes in the skin have the same embryological origin, and previous work (Moore, 2002) has presented experimental evidence to support the hypothetical role of the skin as a large brain. In addition, glia are the other major components of the nervous system, and the morphology of glial cells are very similar to melanocytes.

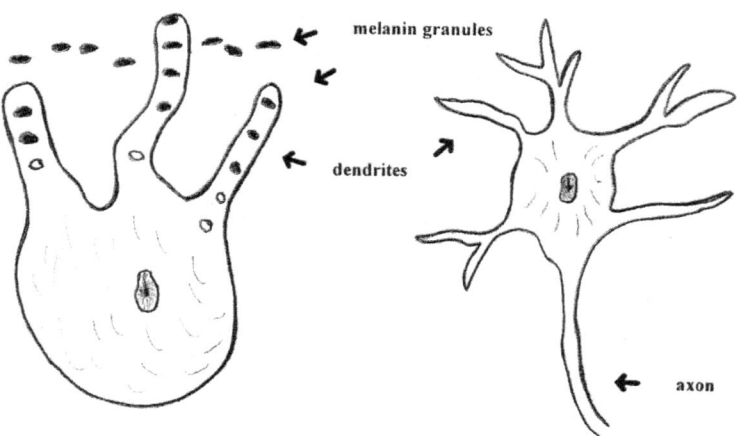

FIG. 1 - *A comparison between the morphology of a skin cell (i.e., melanocyte) and a brain cell (i.e., neuron). Both cell types express dendritic processes that are activated by external stimuli. Both cells secrete chemicals (e.g., melanin for the melanocyte and various types of neurotransmitters for the neuron).*

Moreover, melanin migrates to the peripheral nervous system where the nervous system is in direct contact with the external world via the autonomic nervous system (nerve ganglia connecting all internal organs) and the somatic nervous system (musculature). The endocrine system, which secretes various hormones, is also dependent upon melanin for its structure and function. Furthermore, the nerves for olfaction, vision and hearing are all formed from the presence of melanin, and neurons in these areas contain melanin granules in their cytoplasm. Melanin in all of these regions of the human body can help to provide Aextrasensory@ perceptive abilities. Life is the experience of perceiving what nature has to offer, and experimental research on the biophysical properties of melanin suggests that the experience can be enhanced by the presence of melanin. To clarify this latter point, conceptualize the following three factual scenarios: 1) the absence of pigment in the inner ear would produce deafness; 2) the absence of pigment in the retina would make us virtually blind; and 3) without pigment in specific midbrain brain structures, our psychomotor abilities would be severely impaired. Next, we will review the location of neuromelanin in specific brain structures.

LOCATION OF NEUROMELANIN

The distribution of melanin in the human brain has been mapped by numerous investigators (Olszewski and Baxter, 1954; Olszewski, 1964; Bazelon, et al., 1967; Fenichel and Bazelon, 1968; Graham, 1979; Van Woert, Prasad and Borg, 1967; Sapper and Petito, 1982; Bogerts, 1981), and the cells are primarily located in the brainstem and the midbrain.

Bogerts (1981) studied the brains of four adults (ages 47, 53, 54 and 56) and demonstrated a striking similarity between the location of melanin and the catecholamine cell bodies described in various animal and human fetuses. From the brain areas that were studied, cell counts from the center of each area showed that the mean density of melanin-containing cell bodies were varied considerably between the different areas. Another significant finding from this study was that neuromelanin was not found in the dopamine mesolimbic pathway which is responsible for the reward or pleasure circuit extending from the ventral tegmentum to the nucleus accumbens. This lack of neuromelanin in the reward pathway was surprising because of the concept that both neuromelanin and catecholamines are commonly derived. Others have reported similar findings with a rat that was genetically-sensitive to dopamine (Rot et al., 1995). There were changes in the nigrostriatal dopamine system but not the mesolimbic dopamine system. These are intriguing findings because the great majority of catecholamine melanin-containing cells are dopaminergic (Breathnach, 1988). It is known that melanin is deposited in neurons which are most active in catecholamine synthesis, and the accumulation begins early in life and increases as the animal ages. Hence, neuromelanin may be a marker of active catecholamine metabolism (Fenichel and Bazelon, 1968).

The distribution of melanin-pigmented neurons in human brain closely corresponds to that of catecholamine cell groups in brain of other species (Breathnach, 1988). Furthermore, there are species differences in neuromelanin-containing cells, with guinea pigs and rabbits having none, rat, cat, and dog, some, higher primates more than lower, and man with the most of all (Breathnach, 1988). There are also differences in age distribution in man (Mann and Yates, 1983; Marsden, 1983), and these differences suggest that neuromelanin is not toxic per se, or just an end-product from the biosynthesis of catecholamines.

Early reports suggested that pigmentation was not found in substantia nigra of rabbit, rat, mouse, guinea pig or of most marsupials (Marsden, 1961). In addition, intensity is age dependent since pigmentation was lacking in the substantia nigra of young animals though melanin granules were reported in the human locus coeruleus as early as the fifth month of gestation (Foley and Baxter, 1958). Other than age as a likely factor that can reveal differences in the level of neuromelanin, it is a very significant point to mention how ethnic differences are overlooked when evaluating the presence of neuromelanin. If the claim is made that brain melanin is programmed to function at different capacities depending upon a person=s overall genetic capacity to produce melanin, then it is likely that brain melanin can vary between ethnic groups (Moore, 1995).

The distribution of melanin-pigmented neurons in the human brain was plotted using the brains of three adults (68 to 80 years of age) (Saper and Petito, 1982). These neurons were found primarily in areas corresponding to the A1-A14 catecholamine cell groups which have been reported in other species (Dahlstrom and Fuxe, 1964; Garver and Sladek, 1975). The cells from A1 in the reticular formation extend through the brainstem and midbrain to the A14 cell groups in the hypothalamus (Saper et al., 1982). In another display of the cytoarchitecture of the human brainstem, Olszweski and Baxter (1954) mapped 12 neuromelanin cell groups which can be found in Table I. The substanstia nigra and the locus coeruleus are the two major neuromelanin-containing cell groups. The substantia nigra produces dopamine and the locus coeruleus produces norepinephrine. To provide a visual representation of the location of neuromelanin, Fig. 2 is an illustration of the defined area of the substantia nigra and the locus coeruleus in the brain of a rat immunocytochemically stained for tyrosine hydroxylase. Tyrosine hydroxylase is an enzyme involved in the biosynthesis of catecholamines.

There is another prominent structure called the red nucleus in the midbrain area that is visually distinct as a collection of pigmented neurons. In brief, the red nuclei on the left- and the right-side of the midbrain send axons across the midline of the brainstem into the spinal cord. From the red nucleus to the spinal cord is called the rubrospinal tract, and experimental evidence has demonstrated that this system plays a significant role during voluntary movements of the arm, hand and fingers (Squire, Bloom, McConnell, Roberts, Spitzer and Zigmond, 2003). In Chapter 3, the significance of the red nucleus, and a fully detailed account of these "mirror" neurons will be presented by Adams.

In the next section, we will briefly explore whether or not there is a role for catecholamines in the biosynthesis of neuromelanin.

TABLE 1 - 12 Neuromelanin Cell Groups in the Human Brain Stem Mapped by Olszewski and Baxter (1954) using the Nissl staining technique. <u>Cytoarchitecture of the human brain stem</u>. S. Karger: New York.

1.	**SUBSTANTIA NIGRA (SN)** - Dopamine-containing cells
2.	Nucleus parabrachialis
3.	Nucleus paranigralis
4.	**LOCUS COERULEUS (LC)** - Norepinephrine-containing cells
5.	Nuclei intracapsularis
6.	Subceruleus
7.	Nervi trigemini mesencephalius
8.	Pontis centralis oralis
9.	Tegmenti pedunculopontinus
10.	Parabrachialis medialis
11.	Dorsomotor
12.	Retroambigualis

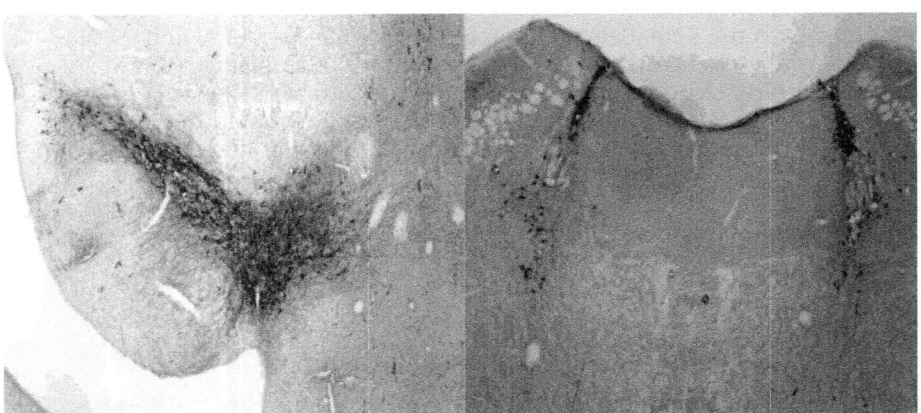

FIG. 2 - *An immunocytochemical technique was used to stain for tyrosine hydroxylase in the substantia nigra (left view) and the locus coeruleus (right view) of a rat brain. The collective group of neurons in each nucleus reveals a distinct section of the brain that would contain neuromelanin.*

BIOSYNTHESIS OF NEUROMELANIN

The biosynthesis of neuromelanin is a fascinating phenomenon because it does not appear to form in the same manner as skin melanin. Skin melanin strictly relies on enzymes (e.g., tyrosinase), whereas little to no evidence supports enzymic activity in pigmented brain cells. For example, Rodgers and Curzon (1975) used a quantitative radiometric assay to compare various substances as melanin precursors in the rat brain. Their goal was to study the ability of different brain regions to form melanin and to evaluate various hypotheses of brain melanin formation. The results of their findings demonstrated that catecholamines, L-DOPA and serotonin were precursors for brain melanin formation. The assay was used to evaluate various hypotheses of brain melanin formation. However, no evidence for enzymic activity was found, and it was concluded that brain melanin formation may be a largely non-enzymic process. Tyrosinase, peroxidase and monoamine oxidase activity were all investigated, and there was minimal to no activity for these enzymes in the brain regions studied. Although enzyme activity appeared to be absent, melanin formation was detected in all brain regions studied and was highest in the substantia nigra and the striatum.

In studies examining the etiology of Parkinson=s Disease (Goldman and Tanner, 1998), the commonly held belief is that neuromelanin is formed by dopamine autoxidation. This concept of autoxidation was proposed by Doyle Graham in 1979. Even with a lack of external melanin, the autoxidation mechanism is a likely explanation for the presence of neuromelanin in a person who lacks substantial amounts of external melanin. However, the inclination is to accept neuromelanin as a waste product of the autoxidation mechanism. In contrast, Barr (1983) stresses the point that neuromelanin is capable of self-synthesis. The self-synthesis hypothesis can buttress the view that neuromelanin is genetically programmed to function at a different capacity depending upon a person=s overall genetic capacity to produce melanin in the body (Moore, 1995).

GENETICS AND NEURODEGENRATIVE DISORDERS

The human genome project has provided valuable information related to diseases that manifest in humans. From current genetics research, there is strong evidence linking genetic abnormalities to the development of neurodegenerative disorders such as Parkinson's disease (PD) and Alzheimer's disease (AD). For example, mutations in the alpha-synuclein gene is implicated in PD (Singleton et al., 2003). Alpha-synuclein was identified as a major component of Lewy bodies, the pathological hallmark of PD, and glial cytoplasmic inclusions (Tu et al., 1998). A similar disease process may resemble the etiology of AD in Down's Syndrome, where expression of the amyloid precursor protein (APP) gene due to chromosome 21 trisomy is the event (Monsonego and Weiner, 2003).

The pathology associated with both PD and AD may be associated with the accumulation of toxic substances that accumulate over years. In AD, amyloid beta-peptide is a cleavage product of neuronal APP. Genetic factors such as APP or presenilin mutations or carrying of the ApoE4 allele results in earlier accumulation of amyloid beta-peptide and early onset of clinical symptoms (Monsonego et al., 2003). In both PD and AD, it is unclear what crucial factors in aging trigger the accumulation of toxic substances in the brain.

In sum, a person can have a genetic predisposition to develop neurodegenerative diseases if there are deficient genetic mechanisms that are unavailable to ward off the accumulation of neurotoxic substances. If a person has a proclivity to develop a neurodegenerative disease, then several factors (e.g., age, diet, toxic exposure) may help to trigger the destruction of neurons. Therefore, it is hypothesized that neuromelanin is genetically programmed to enhance neural functioning by protecting the brain from toxic assaults that accumulate from years of slow poisoning.

NEUROMELANIN AND ETHNICITY

For obvious reasons, it is not possible to dissect the brain of a normal human in order to explore how neuromelanin functions, but the biophysical properties of synthetic melanin in the laboratory can shed light on how neuromelanin is functioning in the brain. Also, experimental evidence can be gathered from animal experiments, pharmacogenetic effects of drugs in patients, and post-mortem analysis of brain tissue.

Racial classifications have historically used skin pigmentation as the sole factor in making a distinction between groups of people. The different levels of skin pigmentation are due to enzymes (e.g., tyrosinase) that determine the amount of melanin that is produced on the external surface of the body. There is no controversy to discuss ethnic differences in skin melanin, but it becomes problematic to discuss ethnic variations in brain melanin. Nearly two decades ago, Lawson (1986) raised the issue about racial and ethnic factors in psychiatric research. There was no direct correlation with melanin or neuromelanin however. We are raising the issue in this book, and as previously stated (Moore,1995), brain melanin is genetically programmed to function at a different capacity depending upon a person's overall genetic capacity to produce melanin.

While the internal molecular arrangements and diffuse interconnections of one=s neuromelanin-catecholamine network may vary uniquely with each individual, such a variation in one=s neuromelanin does not correlate (in any obvious way) with one=s skin color (whether white, red, yellow, black, brown, or albino) (Barr, 1983). A special character of brain melanin is suggested by the normal pigmentation of the substantia nigra and locus coeruleus of albinos who lack melanin pigments elsewhere (Foley and Baxter, 1958). Another intriguing characteristic is the absence of reports of melanomas of these pigmented brain regions even though melanomas of other melanized tissues are well known (Curzon, 1975). To make sense of these anomalous observations, Barr (1983) reminds us that most studies on neuromelanin have been with synthetic melanin *in vitro*. He further states that definitive studies should be done *in vivo* (Barr, 1983).

Definitive studies would help to do away with the concept that neuromelanin is only a waste product. It is the opinion of this author that the waste product terminology should be discarded for two specific reasons: 1) it implies there is no significant value for neuromelanin; and 2) it implies that neuromelanin should be the end-product formed everywhere catecholamines are in high concentration. The first point will be addressed in the next section to emphasize the multiple advantages of neuromelanin functioning. The latter point pertains to enzyme activity which other reports have addressed (Curzon, 1975). Other factors must play a determining factor for the presence of neuromelanin, and the field of genetics can provide clues. Moreover, the biochemistry of melanin/neuromelanin may be the critical factor linked to any genetic variations in the manifestation of psychiatric disorders.

For example, Lawson (1986) has brought to our attention that racial and ethnic differences exist in the symptom presentations of psychiatric disorders. In addition, clinical issues have been raised (Lawson, 1996) to suggest that African Americans have poorer outcomes than Caucasians in general health and mental health systems possibly due to lesser access to services, particularly psychopharmacology in mental health systems. There was only a suggestion that these problems may be exacerbated by ethnic differences in pharmacokinetics (Lawson,1996a; 1996b).

A research team in the Netherlands has uncovered some revealing findings that connect genetics and neural sensitivity in rats (Rot et. al., 1995). Although it is an animal experiment, the data can indirectly support the claim in this chapter that neuromelanin is genetically programmed to function differently depending upon the amount of melanin produced by the individual. In this experiment, pharmacogenetically selected Wistar rat lines were used to investigate the implication of either high or low responsiveness of the dopamine system for the activity of the hypothalamic-pituitary-adrenal (HPA) axis. Apomorphine, a dopamine agonist, was the pharmacological agent used to measure differences between apomorphine-susceptible rats (apo-sus) and apomorphine unsusceptible rats (apo-unsus). The findings revealed increased binding of the dopamine antagonist iodosulpiride to D1/D3 receptors and increased D1 and D2 receptors and mRNA expression in the striatum of apo-sus rats. Moreover, apo-sus rats expressed higher tyrosine hydroxylase mRNA levels in the substantia nigra pars compacta. Collectively, these markers suggested a higher biosynthetic capacity of dopamine in the nigrostriatal pathway and a higher responsiveness of the striatal dopamine receptors. This potentially enhanced reactivity of the nigrostriatal dopamine system coincides with the much higher sensitivity of these rats to apomorphine-induced stereotypic behavior.

In addition, the authors demonstrated a genetic link between dopamine susceptibility and stress-induced HPA activation. For example, their findings suggested that increased susceptibility of the dopamine system, and increased tyrosine hydroxylase mRNA and D2/D3 receptor capacity coincides with increased central HPA drive and corticosteroid feedback resistance. Since it was demonstrated that there are differences in neuroendocrine response patterns against a dopamine-dependent genetic background, it is hypothesized that individual differences in dopamine are linked to the magnitude and duration of HPA activation. In other words, a more sensitive dopamine system can help an individual effectively deal with stress. The dopamine system is activated during stress to release HPA hormones, but overactivation may lead to negative physiological consequences. The high incidence of stroke, hypertension and other cardiovascular imbalances could result from an overly sensitive dopamine system that impacts the neuromelanin-catecholamine network.

Ethnobiological differences in response to drugs have been observed with both psychoactive or mind-altering drugs (Lin, Poland and Chien, 1990; Strickland, Lin, Fu, Anderson and Zheng, 1995; Wood and Zhou, 1991) as well as nonpsychoactive drugs (Flaherty and Meagher, 1980). Strickland and Gray (2000) explored the significance of ethnobiological variation in drug responsivity to drugs that are known to treat mood disorders such as depression, anxiety and schizophrenia. Many of the drugs that have been developed to treat mental disorders affect neurotransmitter systems that come from melinated centers in the brain. For example, norepinephrine, serotonin and dopamine are neurotransmitters involved in mood disorders and each neurochemical is produced from specific brain nuclei that are visibly melinated. Interestingly, it has been reported that African Americans have a higher risk of developing tardive dyskinesia than Caucasians, even when differences in neuroleptic drug use are accounted for (Eastham, Lacro and Jeste, 1996). Asians appeared to have a lower or equal risk of developing tardive dyskinesia compared with Caucasians.

Even though scientists claim that the amount of neuromelanin is independent of skin melanin, there is reason to believe that there could be variations in the sensitivity of neuromelanin functioning. Everyone has skin covering their bodies, but there are some people who are more sensitive to touch. Everyone has eyes to see, but some people are more sensitive to certain types of light. Everyone has ears, but some people are more sensitive to specific kinds of frequencies of sound. Likewise, one can have a genetic predisposition for a more sensitive neuromelanin-catecholamine network.

Parkinson=s Disease

Parkinson=s Disease (PD) is a neurodegenerative disease that mostly affects the elderly. PD is pathologically characterized by destruction of dopaminergic cells in the midbrain region called the substantia nigra. The substantia nigra is a highly melinated subcortical structure. As part of the basal ganglia (motor system), it has an integral role in regulating and producing slow coordinated and deliberate movements. Besides destruction of substantia nigra neurons, there is also degeneration of cells in the ventral tegmentum and the locus coeruleus (Kaplan and Sadock, 1987). The combined effect of this neurodegeneration leads to tremor, muscle rigidity, bradykinesia (slow movements), stooped posture and a shuffling gait. By observing the psychomotor impairments of neurodegenerative disorders such as PD, one can infer how the brain controls normal behavior.

A thorough investigation of the behavioral impairments and motor deficits associated with PD can indirectly reveal how the substantia nigra functions. It can be speculated that a highly melinated substantia nigra can produce advanced motor skills throughout the lifetime of the organism. As the individual ages, the presence of neuromelanin increases, but there may be a loss of catecholamine neurons in the melinated brain region. Age-related reasons have been the primary factor attributing to the development of PD; however, there are numerous cases of PD-like symptoms in young people who have experimented with drugs. In the 1970s there was a connection between a synthetic drug called MPTP and thirty years later there is a connection with another designer drug called Ecstasy. Therefore, age is not the only etiology for PD. The drug effects on the pigmented neurons in the brain suggest that the biophysical properties of neuromelanin can contribute to the destruction of these specialized cells that are primarily involved in psychomotor tasks.

The effects of these designer drugs in young people have led some to believe that there are environmental risk factors associated with PD. Marder and colleagues (1998) used univariate and multivariate unconditional logistic regression models in 89 nondemented patients with PD and 188 control subjects in a multiethnic urban community. Rural living, area farming, and drinking well water were associated with PD only in African Americans. In Hispanics, area farming was protective, whereas drinking unfiltered water was a risk factor for PD. The authors concluded that ethnic and cultural origin may add to the epidemiological study of PD.

There has been a suggestion that people of African descent are less likely to develop PD when compared to other ethnic groups. For example, the large-scale pattern of underlying-cause PD mortality among whites has persisted for three decades (Lanska, 1997). Lanska used the National Center for Health Statistics and Bureau of the Census to map age-adjusted, race- and race-gender-specific PD mortality rates in the U.S. for 1998. Reported rates among blacks were significantly lower than among whites. Among whites, high underlying-cause rates predominated in the North and low rates predominated in the South.

In 1993, Gilbert analyzed the low risk of aging Africans as opposed to high risk Caucasians to certain major disorders. The disorders included PD, myocardial infarction, osteoporosis and fractures, some rheumatic diseases, and an overall reduced incidence of cancer. In this European-based study, the relative risk was determined by a common physiological mechanism involving the autonomic nervous system and calcium metabolism. In addition, increased vagal tone, enhanced dopaminergic activity, an efficient dopamine/vitamin D-parathormone system and a neuroendocrine-metabolic context may determine the response to specific stimuli. As speculated from the previously mentioned genetic sensitivity study with rats (Rot et al., 1995), Gilbert suggested that maintained dopaminergic activity, as proposed for Africans, coupled with low risk to certain disorders, confirms the experimentally demonstrated paramount importance of this neurotransmitter in retarding aging processes in animals. The neuroendocrine profiles as defined for Africans is consistent with a potentially extended period of physical and mental competence and a conceivable shorter duration of involuntary decline (Gilbert, 1993).

In another epidemiological study, Kurtzke and Goldberg (1988) reported that age-adjusted death rates for PD in the U.S. from 1959 to 1961 demonstrated significantly lower rates for blacks than for whites, with rates for Asian Americans the same as for whites. In another study (de la Monte, Hutchins and Moore, 1989), it was determined that the dementia due to PD was more frequent among whites, the frequencies of multi-infarct dementia and dementia due to chronic ethanol abuse were higher among blacks, and the frequency of Alzheimer=s disease was 2.6 times higher among whites. The study explored racial differences in the etiology of

Alzheimer=s disease and a strong argument was made in favor of a genetic transmission of sporadic Alzheimer=s disease.

Some studies report that blacks have a lower rate of developing PD than Caucasians, whereas some studies have not found such a difference. For instance, a review conducted by Richards and Chaudhuri (1996) reported that the confounding effects may be due to a low case ascertainment and high selective mortality. Even though people of African origin may be more protected from the effects of PD, there is data to suggest that people of African descent are vulnerable to vascular PD, which is associated with high mortality. Moreover, lower life expectancy and failure of old people to attend hospitals in South Africa may be factors in the apparent low prevalence of PD among blacks (Cosnett and Bill, 1988).

A study performed in India (Muthane, Yasha and Shankar, 1998) further supports the ethnic variation in neuromelanin that has been reiterated in this chapter. The objectives of this study were to count the number of melanized neurons in the substantia nigra pars compacta in normal human brains from India and study the change in neuronal count with advancing age and to compare the neuronal counts from this Indian population with counts reported in normal brains from the United Kingdom (UK). In the brains from India, there was no loss of melanized nigral neurons with advancing age. The absolute number of these melanized neurons was about 40% lower than the brains from UK. Despite a low number of melanized nigral neurons in the brains from India, individuals function normally and have dopamine levels comparable with their Western counterparts. Therefore, it is not the absolute number of melanized nigral neurons that solely attributes to the development of PD. There is no significant loss of pigmented nigral neurons with age, suggesting that the loss seen in PD is exclusively due to the disease process itself. The authors concluded that Indians have a lower prevalence of PD despite having a low count of melanized nigral neurons, suggesting that better protective mechanisms may be present in the Indians to prevent the loss of nigral neurons.

According to Chaudhuri, Hu and Brooks (2000), ongoing studies in India suggest that the pattern of PD tends to differ from Afro-Caribbean subjects in the UK. These authors are attempting to unravel the mechanism of increased frequency of atypical PD in these ethnic groups and include genetic studies addressing polymorphisms of enzymes metabolizing levodopa, dietary neurotoxin screening and functional imaging studies of the striatum using positron emission tomography. As we have discussed earlier, cardiovascular challenges such as diabetes and hypertension are being considered as significant factors affecting people of African descent.

In sum, there is substantial evidence to support the claim that neuromelanin may function differently depending upon biochemistry and a person=s overall genetic capacity to produce melanin. Animal experiments exploring genetics and neural sensitivity, ethnobiological variations in response to drug effects, and the higher incidence rate of PD in non-Black people suggests that neuromelanin has a functional role in the nervous system.

ADVANTAGES OF NEUROMELANIN

We commonly think of melanin as a photoprotective pigment in the skin that can block the damaging effects of ultraviolet radiation (UVR) from the sun. UVR is an external stimulus, and it does not reach the inner depths of the brain. Therefore, it is difficult to comprehend why melanin is found deep in the brain if it is not due to stimulation from the sun. Most of the speculation on the significance of neuromelanin formation has resulted from studies on neurodegeneration of pigmented brain neurons or from studies of synthetic melanin in the laboratory. The clueless adventure has slowly faded as we have gained more knowledge concerning the biophysical properties of melanin.

Toxic Neutralizer

Melanin is effective as a device for radiation-less conversion of the energy of harmfully excited molecules into innocuous vibrational energy (McGinness and Proctor, 1973). This conversion may deactivate metabolically excited molecules that can become potentially damaging to cells. Since there are no mechanical devices involved, that is why this conversion is called radiation-less. The important point is that melanin helps to ensure that the spread of further cellular damage is neutralized.

Melanin is also known to protect against dangerous free radicals. Free radicals are highly reactive chemical species that have an odd number of electrons, and hence, one unpaired electron. It has been proposed (Commoner, Townsend and Pake, 1954) that melanin acts like a deposit site or sink for unpaired electrons, thus removing reactive free radicals. Peroxides are examples of chemical substances that can lose an electron and change into dangerous and cytotoxic substances.

Besides cytotoxic molecules and free radicals, melanin has a redox capacity to prevent Arust@ in the brain. For example, if you leave iron in water, it will oxidize and rust. In the body, melanin can act as an electron-transfer agent to protect cells and tissue against reducing or oxidizing conditions (van Woert, 1968; Gan, 1976; 1977). By assisting in the transfer of electrons, melanin ensures the safe conversion of potentially volatile chemical reactions.

Nerve Conduction Facilitator

Ions are charged particles that we consume in our diets in the form of electrolytes. When dissolved in water, these electrolytes can conduct an electrical current. These electrolytes set up a weak biological current in the nervous system that ranges from 40 to 120 millivolts that can be harnessed by melanin (McGinness, Cory and Proctor, 1974). Melanin can act as a threshold switch to change the voltage for neuronal firing. In other words, there is more activity elicited from melinated brain regions when compared to nonmelinated brain regions.

It was first suggested by McGinness in 1972 that melanin may act as an amorphous semiconductor since there is a rise in the conductivity of melanin under an applied voltage. McGinness suggested that this rise might be a result of increased kinetic energy of the electrons leading to higher mobility and promotion to excited states.

It is suggested that the bioelectronic properties associated with melanin can help to facilitate nerve conduction in the following three ways: 1) it can speed the pace of the nerve impulse; 2) it can concentrate ions for high voltage generating activity; and 3) it can provide an electrochemical surge.

In the context of mental health, melinated cells can cause a greater release of neurochemicals from nerve cells. Neural transmission requires the stimulation of certain electrolytes across the cell membrane. As a result of this change in the cell membrane, neurochemicals are released from the cell to transmit a nerve impulse. As we previously discussed, there are several brain regions (e.g., substantia nigra, locus coeruleus, raphe nucleus) that have both high melanin content and neurochemical activity (e.g., dopamine, norepinephrine, serotonin). Therefore, neuromelanin can increase the voltage, cause an electrochemical surge, and positively influence the release of neurochemicals.

Energy Transformer

The consistent appearance of melanin in living organisms at locations where energy conversion or charge transfer occurs (e.g., skin, retina, inner ear) is of particular interest. Melanin is strategically located in the body to absorb and to convert various forms of electromagnetic energy into energy states that can be used by the nervous system. Essentially, it can function as an electrochemical transducer.

The fact that melanin is black or dark in color could help explain how it functions as a converter of energy. Since dark skin or any black substance absorbs heat, light is not reradiated, but is converted to rotational and vibrational degrees of freedom (McGinness and Proctor, 1973). Contrary to blackness, whiteness reflects light. As a result, pigmented cells are more capable of converting energy versus nonpigmented cells. Although there appears to be comparable distributions of neuromelanin in the brain when compared between ethnic groups, darker colored people have a more modified external pigmentary system that has a greater capacity for charge transfer.

At the level of the brain cell, however, there are significant neurophysiological functions that are constantly improving the excitation and conductivity of the nervous system. Stimulation of the nervous system requires an action potential and any change in the electronic nature of the neuromelanin could generate vibrational energy capable of affecting nerve impulses. Action potentials are generated when ions or electrolytes flow in and out of the cell membrane. When physical stimuli from the outside world is converted into neural impulses, neuromelanin could act as a semiconductor to increase the firing rate of action potentials.

BIOLOGICAL ACTIVATION OF NEUROMELANIN

Neuromelanin is a potent antioxidant. To biologically activate neuromelanin, it is important to ingest the proper nutritional items to promote the functioning of the neuromelanin-catecholamine network. Current research has documented the protective role of pigments in certain fruits that can function as effective antioxidants. For example, black berries and blue berries are at the top of the list of fruits that function as effective antioxidants. Interestingly, the darker the berry - the greater the antioxidant effect. Since neuromelanin has a protective role as an effective antioxidant, a person=s health can be greatly enhanced by consuming substances that have a similar role in health promotion.

It is essential to consume as many natural food items as possible to decrease the chances of developing neurodegenerative diseases as Professor will elaborate in the next chapter. The accumulation of toxic chemicals and artificial substances over the years can be absorbed by the pigmented neurons in the brain and lead to cellular damage. The antioxidant properties found in many fruits can slow the aging process and prevent cellular damage. In addition, studies on the effects of blueberries have demonstrated that these dark berries can improve cognitive skills and motor performance in rats (Joseph, Nadeau and Underwood, 2002).

In sum, there are many sun-enriched products (e.g., fruits and vegetables) that have natural chemical substances that are necessary for the nervous system to function at an optimal level. Vitamins, minerals, amino acids and alkaloids are a few of the substances that can biologically activate neuromelanin and promote positive physical and mental health.

CONCLUSION

Neuromelanin can be considered the core of consciousness. It is the connection between the blackness of interstellar space (dark matter) and the pigment deep within the recesses of our nervous system (neuromelanin) that we can begin to contemplate a new way of thinking about consciousness. As we have reviewed in this chapter, the presence of neuromelanin increases from lower to higher animals and it is highest in man. When comparing the conscious awareness of other species, man is usually placed at the top of the list.

The unique display of flamboyant expressiveness in African/Black culture is primarily due to a highly energized sensory-motor network. The expressiveness can be displayed in rhythmically-oriented tasks such a dancing, rapping to a beat, moving the body to a percussive rhythm, and nearly all tasks involving psychomotor skills. Beyond skill development, Bynum in Chapter 3 and King in Chapter 4 will further discuss the role of neuromelanin in mental processes or what we know as consciousness. They have placed neuromelanin as a central theme in their explorations of mind and human consciousness (King, 1990; Bynum, 1999).

From a biological perspective, the presence of neuromelanin can be a double-edged sword. It can protect the brain as well as lead to damaging alterations in brain cells. On the one hand, a properly functioning neuromelanin-catecholamine network can greatly enhance a person=s psychomotor abilities, but any impairment of these pigmented neurons can cause neurodegenerative diseases such as Parkinson=s disease. To conclude, neuromelanin is not a waste product. Neuromelanin is critical to maintaining a healthy state of mind. To promote positive mental health, it is encouraged to consume as many natural products to stimulate the antioxidant, semiconductive and electrochemical transducing properties of neuromelanin.

REFERENCES

Barr, F.E. (1983). Melanin: the organizing molecule. Medical Hypothesis, 11(1), 1-140.

Bazelon, M., Fenichel, G.M. and Randall, J. (1967). Studies on neuromelanin. I. a melanin system in the human adult brainstem. Neurology, 17, 512-519.

Bogerts, B. (1981). A brainstem atlas of catecholaminergic neurons in man, using melanin as a natural marker. Journal of Comparative Neurology, 197, 63-80.

Breathnach, A.S. (1988). Extra-cutaneous melanin. Pigment Cell Research, 1, 234-237.

Bynum, E.B. (1999). African Unconscious: Roots of Ancient Mysticism and Modern Psychology. New York: Teachers College Press.

Chaudhuri, K.R., Hu, M.T. and Brooks, D.J. (2000). Atypical parkinsonsism in Afro-Caribbean and Indian origin immigrants to the UK. Movement Disorders, 15(1), 18-23.

Clark, C., McGee, D.P., Nobles, W. and Weems, L. (1975). Voodoo or I.Q.: An introduction to African psychology. Journal of Black Psychology, 1(2), 9-29.

Commoner, B., Townsend, J. and Pake G.E. (1954). Free radicals in biological materials. Nature, 174, 689-691.

Cosnett, J.E. and Bill, P.L. (1988). Parkinson=s disease in blacks. Observations on epidemiology in Natal. South African Medical Journal, 73(5), 281-283.

Curzon, G. (1975). Metals and melanins in the extrapyramidal centers. Pharmacological Therapeutics Bulletin, 1(4), 673-684.

Dahlstrom, A. and Fuxe, K. (1964). Evidence for the existence of monoamine-containing neurons in the central nervous system. I. Demonstration of monoamines in the cell bodies of brain stem neurons. Acta Physiologica Scandinavica, 62, Supplement 232, 1-55.

de la Monte, S.M., Hutchins, G.M. and Moore, G.W. (1989). Racial differences in the etiology of dementia and frequency of Alzheimer lesions in the brain. Journal of the National Medical Association, 81(6), 644-52.

de Montellano, B.R.O. (1993). Melanin, afrocentricity, and pseudoscience. Yearbook of Physical Anthropology, 36, 33-58.

Eastham, J.H., Lacro, J.P. and Jeste, D.V. (1996). Ethnicity and movement disorders. Mount Sinai Journal of Medicine, 63(5-6), 314-319.

Fenichel, G.M. and Bazelon, M. (1968). Studies on neuromelanin. II. melanin in the brainstems of infants and children. Neurology, 18, 817-820.

Flaherty, J.A. and Meagher, R. (1980). Measuring racial bias in inpatient treatment. American Journal of Psychiatry, 127, 679-682.

Foley, J.M. and Baxter,D. (1958). On the nature of pigment granules in the cells of the locus coeruleus and substantia nigra. Journal of Neuropathology and Experimental Neurology, 17, 586-598.

Gan, E.V., Haberman, H.F. and Menon, I.A. (1976). Electron transfer properties of melanin. <u>Archives in Biochemisry and Biophysics, 173</u>, 666-672.

Gan, E.V., Lam, K.M., Haberman, H.F. and Menon, I.A. (1977). Electron transfer properties of melanins. <u>British Journal of Dermatology, 96</u>, 25-28.

Garver, D.L. and Sladek, J.R. (1975). Monoamine distribution in primate brain. I. Catecholamine-containing perikarya in the brain stem of *Macaca speciosa*. <u>Journal of Comparative Neurology, 159</u>, 289-304.

Gilbert, C. (1993). Low risk to certain diseases in aging: role of the autonomic nervous system and calcium metabolism. <u>Mechanisms of Ageing and Development, 70</u>(1-2), 95-113.

Goldman, S.M. and Tanner, C. (1998). Etiology of parkinson=s disease. In J Jankovic and E. Tolosa (Eds.). <u>Parkinson=s Disease and Movement Disorders (3rd Ed.)</u> 133-158. Baltimore, MD: Lippincott, Williams and Wilkins.

Graham, D.G. (1978). Oxidative pathways for catecholamines in the genesis of neuromelanin and cytotoxic quinones. <u>Molecular Pharmacology, 14</u>, 633-643.

Graham, D.G. (1979). On the origin and significance of neuromelanin. <u>Archives in Pathological Laboratory Medicine, 103</u>, 359-362.

Hannaford, C. (1995). Smart Moves: Why Learning Is Not All In Your Head. Alexander, NC: Great Ocean Publishers.

Joseph, J., Nadeau, D. and Underwood, A. (2002). The Color Code: A revolutionary eating plan for optimum health. New York: Hyperion.

Kaplan, H.I. and Sadock, B.J. (1988). <u>Synopsis of Psychiatry: Behavioral Sciences Clinical Psychiatry</u> (5th ed.). Baltimore: Williams and Wilkins.

King, R. (1990). African Origin of Biological Psychiatry. Tennessee: Seymour-Smith Inc.

Kurtzke, J.F. and Goldberg, I.D. (1988). Parkinsonism death rates by race, sex, and geography. Neurology, 38(10), 1558-61.

Lanska, D.J. (1997). The geographic distribution of parkinson=s disease mortality in the United States. Journal of Neurological Science, 150(1), 63-70.

Lawson, W.B (1986). Racial and ethnic factors in psychiatric research. Hospital Community Psychiatry, Jan, 37(1), 50-4.

Lawson, W.B. (1996a). Clinical issues in the pharmacotherapy of African-Americans. Pharmacological Bulletin, 32(2), 275-281.

Lawson, W.B. (1996b). The art and science of the psychopharmacotherapy of African Americans. Mt. Sinai Journal of Medicine, Oct.-Nov., 63(5-6), 301-05.

Le Douarin, N.M. and Kalcheim, C. (1999). The Neural Crest. New York: Cambridge University Press.

Lin, K.M., Poland, R.E. and Chien, C.P. (1990). Ethnicity and psychopharmacology: Recent findings and future research directions. In E. Sorel (Ed.), Family, Culture and Psychobiology. New York: Legas.

Mann, D.M.A. and Yates, P.O. (1983). Possible role of neuromelanin in the pathogenesis of Parkinson's disease. Mechanisms in Age Development, 21, 193-203.

Marder, K., Logroscino, G., Alfaro, B., Mejia, H., Halim, A., Louis, E., Cote, L. and Mayeux, R. (1998). Environmental risk factors for parkinson=s disease in an urban multiethnic community. Neurology, 50(1), 279-281.

Marsden, C.D. (1961). Pigmentation in the nucleus substantia nigra of mammals. Journal of Anatomy, 95, 256-261.

Marsden, C.D. (1983). Neuromelanin and parkinson's disease. Journal of Neural Transmission, 19, 121-141.

McGinness, J. (1972). Mobility gaps: A mechanism for band gaps in melanins. Science, 177, 896.

McGinness, J. and Proctor, P. (1973). The importance of the fact that melanin is black Journal of Theoretical Biology, 39, 677-688.

McGinness, J., Corry, P. and Proctor, P. (1974). Amorphous semiconductor switching in melanins. Science, 183, 853-855.

Monsonego, A. and Weiner, H.L. (2003). Immunotherapuetic approaches to Alzheimer's disease. Science, 302(5646), 834-838.

Moore, T.O. (1995). The Science of Melanin: Dispelling the Myths. Silver Spring, MD: Beckham House Publishers.

Moore, T.O. (2002). Dark Matters Dark Secrets. Redan, GA: Zamani Press.

Muthane, U., Yasha, T.C. and Shankar, S.K. (1998). Low numbers and no loss of melanized nigral neurons with increasing age in normal human brains from India. Annals in Neurology, 43(3), 283-87.

Olszewski, J. and Baxter, D. (1954). Cytoarchitecture of the human brain stem. Basel: S. Karger.

Olszewski, J. (1964). Cytoarchitecture of the Human Brain. New York: Stern and Birjelow.

Oppenheimer, S,B. and Lefevre, G. (1984). Introduction to Embryonic Development. Massachusettes: Allyn and Bacon, Inc.
Reichardt, L.F. and Farinas, I. (1999). Early actions of neurotrophic factors. In M. Sieber-Blum
(Ed.). Neurotrophins and the Neural Crest (pp. 1-27). Boca Raton, FL: CRC Press.

Richards, M. and Chaudhuri, K.R. (1996). Parkinson=s disease in populations of African origin: a review. Neuroepidemiology, 15(4), 214-221.

Rodgers, A.D. and Curzon, G. (1975). Melanin formation by human brain in vitro. Journal of Neurochemistry, 24 1123-1129.

Rot et al., (1995). Corticosteriod feedback resistance in rats genetically selected for increased dopamine responsiveness. Journal of Neuroendocrinology, 7, 153-161.

Sapper, C.B. and Petito, C.K. (1982). Correspondence of melanin-pigmented neurons in human brain with A1-A14 catecholamine cell groups. Brain, 105, 87-101.

Singleton, A.B. et al. (2003). Alpha-synuclein locus triplication causes Parkinson's disease. Science, 302(5646), 841.

Squire, L. R., Bloom, F.E., McConnell, S.K., Roberts, J.L., Spitzer, N.C. and Zigmond, M.J. (2003). Fundamental Neuroscience (2nd Ed.). San Diego, CA: Academic Press.

Strickland, T.L., Lin, K.M., Fu, P., Anderson, D. and Zheng, Y. (1995). Comparison of lithium ratio between African American and Caucasian bipolar patients. Society of Biological Psychiatry, 37, 325-330.

Strickland, T.L. and Gray, G. (2000). Neurobehavioral disorders and pharmacologic Intervention.   In E. Fletcher-Janzen, T. Strickland and C.R. Reynolds. Handbook of Cross-Cultural Neuropsychology. pp. 361-369. New York:Kluwer Academic/Plenum Publishers.

Tu et al. (1998). Annals in Neurology, 44, 415.

Van Woert, M.H., Prasad, K.N. and Borg, D.C. (1967). Spectroscopic studies of substantia nigra pigment in human sybjects. Journal of Neurochemisty, 14, 707-716.

Van Woert, M.H. (1968). DPNH oxidation by melanin: inhibition by phenothiazines. Proceedings in Social, Experimental and Biological Medicine, 129, 165-171.

Wood, A.J. and Zhou, H.H. (1991). Ethnic differences in drug disposition and responsiveness. Clinical Pharmacokinetics, 20, 1-24.

CHAPTER 2

NEUROMELANIN: WHAT IS ITS IMPORTANCE IN NEURAL TISSUE?

Ann C. Brown, Ph.D.
Medgar Evers College

OVERVIEW

Melanins are pigmented organic biopolymers found in the biosphere, lithosphere, atmosphere, and the cosmos. In living organisms, it is eumelanin, phaeomelanin and allomelanin. Eumelanin is the polymerization of nitrogenous melanogens; phaeomelamin is derived from the polymerization of sulfurated melanogens; and, allomelanin is the polymerization of polyphenols. In the brain, the black material is referred to as neuromelanin (melanin of neural tissue). A midsagittal section through the human brain exposes the circumventricular organs (CVO), so-called because of their topology around the deep cavities in the brain, all contain neuromelanin in some quantity. Neuromelanin is a macromolecule found in a significant amount in catecholaminergic neurons, especially dopaminergic and noradrenergic neurons in the human brain. Neuromelanin is a brown/black biopolymer pigment found in membrane bound vesicles in the human central nervous system, primarily in the substantia nigra and locus coeruleus. Neuromelanin has been shown to act as a reservoir for the storage of heavy metals, antioxidants, the formation and scavenger of free radicals. The storage of heavy metals and organic toxins have been interpreted as a protective function for neuromelanin. Two dementias of the elderly are Alzheimer's and Parkinson's diseases. Brain researchers found evidence that a protein called ApoE (a lipoprotein E) within nerve cells in the brains of Alzheimer's patients sets off a cascade of biochemical events that decrease and finally destroys neuronal cells in critical areas of the human brain. Studies have shown that in patients with Alzheimer's disorder, a degeneration of synapses and neuronal death, in sections of the brain involved in learning and memory. Clinically, Alzheimer's is manifested as memory loss, and eventually cell death. Parkinson's disease is a slow age-related neurodegenerative disease that results in selective cell death of the neuromelanin pigment producing neuronal cells in the mesencephalic substantia nigra pars compacta and the locus coeruleus. Nevertheless, there are some unanswered questions regarding the role of neuromelanin in Parkinson's disease. Nuclear magnetic resonance spectroscopy and X-ray diffraction studies have shown that neuromelanin is a multilayer, three-dimensional structure, synthesized enzymatically from the conversion of tyrosine to L-DOPA, dopamine, DOPA-quinone via tyrosinase. Neuromelanin than reacts with other macromolecules, such as lipids and proteins and accumulates with age in the neurons as lipofucsin granules in areas of the brain. Finally, neuromelanin is important in all brain functions, and that Parkinson' and Alzheimer's disorders may be different manifestations of the same condition. It appears that most of the brain disorders, to some degree, depend on the neuromelanin via dopamine and acetylcholine needed for motor control, to maintain functional health. There may strong implications of poor nutrition in the etiology of many of the long-term neurological diseases. Other possible roles that neuromelanin may contribute to consciousness, memory and spirituality to maintain healthy behavior are being considered.

Definition

Melanin is precipitated as black material. Black materials are present throughout the universe (Nicolaus 1964, 1965). In the biosphere as eumelanin, phaeomelanin, allomelanin; in the lithosphere as minerals, graphites, fullerenes; in the atmosphere as pollutants, smoke; in the hydrosphere in seas, lakes, rivers; and, in the cosmos as fullerenes, cosmids (Nicolaus, 1964). Melanin is an amorphous semiconductor because it is always in motion, always changing as a result of its central chemical core by adjusting to various energy levels. Because of this motion, melanins display consistent semiconductor properties, by virtue of low resistance to the flow of electrons (Strezelecka, 1982; Riley, 1997; Bynum, 1999). Therefore, melanin serves as a switch for the flow of electrons to higher or lower levels of energy. The low frequency of charge transfer currency renders melanin with the ability to bind with strong affinity to drugs and metals to ultimately damage neural tissue and overall functions via cell death (Swart, 1992; Barnes, 1999).

Its presence in all living organisms has been fully documented and is suggestive of its involvement in many critical functions (perhaps protective) required by all cells to function and maintain life (Lindquist, 1987). Bynum (1999), on the basis of recent experimental data reported in the literature, suggests that neuromelanin may be a superconductor, that is, it appears to have s the capacity to enter into a particular state in which energy is conducted through the system with a high degree of efficiency (Cope, 1971,1978). Bynum further states that these lines of melanin and neuromelanin conductivity in the fetus of the mother's womb are present from the earliest stages of embryogenesis. They are prior to the first heartbeat. In fact, early in embryogenesis there are perceived 'lines of force' that evolve and later may unfold the forms and templates of human cognitive, emotional, and noetic or spiritual experience. In that light, given its bioluminous capacities, its pervasiveness throughout the biological processes, and its crucial significance from the very earliest stages of human life and experience, including life in the womb of the mother, melanin is the chemical of life, the chemical of what our ancestors called the soul, the transformational doorway through which the energy waves of the Holy Soul, Spirit, and Mind pass to take form as the Holy Body. Ancient Africans in the classical literature (*Meter Neter*; James, 1954) and psychology of Kemet (Egypt) (Diop, 1974; Akbar, 1984), viewed all the contents of Amenta (the underworld–personal subconscious (Mind), superconscious (Soul), collective unconscious (Spirit), as jet black in color (King, 1990, 2001). Barr (1983) lists established and proposed properties of melanin that reflect its numerous functions and documents the behavior due to its biophysical and biochemical properties. Barr further advances a major hypothesis that "melanin (in conjunction with other pigment/pigment-related molecules, such as the ubiquitous isopentenoid polymers), functions as the most significant organizational molecule in living systems through its effective *in vivo* control of the vital and diverse covalent current switching." This is a very important concept as it relates to the ability of melanin to generate some degree of low level electrical current in living systems that generates the current needed for nerve conductivity. Given the temperature in brain neural tissue, neuromelanin, as an amorphous semiconductor and superconductor can conceivably transmit electrical current without resistance in such a closed environment as perpetual motion that scientists call a "macroscopic quantum phenomenon" (Nicolaus, 1997). Therefore, nerve cells, for example, are very specialized to receive, process, and transmit information (consciousness) throughout the body in perpetual motion.

    This report advances the hypothesis that neuromelanin (brain melanin) is important in neural tissue to direct and transmit the flow of electrical current via nerve cells (neurons) to all portions of the brain. That flow is tantamount to "consciousness." In effect, neuromelanin is consciousness. Neurons that are deficient in this black material will show a deficit in current energy, thus jeopardizing consciousness, intellect, motor activity and other critical functions. Its presence in all mammalian species and in lower vertebrates has been fully documented and speaks for its importance in living organisms. Our interest in neuromelanin is to express a consolidated theoretical approach as psychiatrists, scientists, and psychologists drawing from the wealth of research, including pathological conditions increasingly diagnosed in the population throughout the world. We realized most of what is known of these pathologies are based on effects, but we must state them, knowing that the causes are always nebulous. Nevertheless, we are also interested in *cause* as well as *effects*. Real answers to pathologies will not be a reality unless causes are first identified. Except for the role of neuromelanin in pathological states (effects), such as seen in Parkinson's and Alzheimer's diseases and certain neurological tumors, past and present interests by investigators of the role of dark pigment concentrated in several strategic areas of the brain and elsewhere have all but been ignored. As a matter of fact, except for the politics of skin melanin, little attention has been given to its significance in nerve functions. Why is it present in the cell body of a neuron? Even today, the nomenclature concerned with neuromelanin is evaded in the investigative efforts, for it is assumed to be just a pigmented cytosolic *waste product* of catecholamine synthesis. However, according to Cotzias (1964): "the neuromelanin granule may be the secret key to the understanding of Parkinsonism. I don't believe God put the melanin granule in the central nervous system (CNS) for nothing. It must be doing something. Something big . . ."

Location and Importance of Neuromelanin

Neuromelanin is a dark pigment that aggregates as granules in the cytoplasm of catecholaminergic neurons in the brainstem (midbrain, pons, and medulla), and the epithelial layers of the ventricles of the brain of humans and has been shown to be different from melanin in skin melanocytes (Mason, 1959; Schraermeyer, 1996; Zecca, 1992). It is particularly high in the *substantia nigra pars compacta* of the midbrain and noradrenergic neurons in the *locus coeruleus* of the fourth ventricle. Neuromelanin tends to accumulate with aging, which links it to certain neurodegenerative diseases (Graham, 1978; Bogerts, 1981). The *locus coeruleus* neuromelanin content has been correlated with feelings of prudence, watchfulness, attentiveness to terror, panic, fear, impulsivity, carelessness and recklessness (King, 1994).

Classical pioneering data are available from a number of scientists to explain much of cellular interactions during development. Fertilization results from melanin-containing female egg (Harsa-King, 1980) and melanin-containing male spermatozoa (Barr, 1983). The sperm entry leaves an electrical pathway of pigment in the frog oocyte (Rugh, 1977; Robinson, 1979). During embryogenesis, a specialized melanized area, Black Dot, (King, 1990) of ectodermal tissue achieve neuronal potential by contact or "primary induction" from the roof of the archenteron (Spemann, 1938). Neural crest forms from this neuroectoderm, folds and separates from the overlying ectoderm to form a neural tube (future spinal cord). Neural crest cells are bilaterally-paired populations of cells arising in the ectoderm at the margins of the neural tube. These pluripotent crest cells migrate away from the neural tube along many pathways to give rise to diverse cell types and derivatives, including sensory and autonomic ganglia, Schwann cells, chromaffin cells, melanocytes, retina, retinal pigmented layer, and many other structures (Weston, 1982; Pavan & Tilghman, 1994). The question becomes, what causes this original homogeneous population of cells to migrate and give rise to these diverse cell types? A number of hypotheses have been proposed. Our hypothesis is that extracellular matrix receptor proteins and intracellular melanin molecules serve as the guiding impetus that give clues via cell-to-cell signaling as *organizing molecules* (as in Barr, 1983). Cohen and Konigsberg (1975), using the avian system, developed a technique to study neural crest cell migration patterns by removing the crest cells and placing them in culture and subsequently replating them to establish clones (single precursor population). They found that three types of clones arose: all pigmented cells, all non-pigmented cells and a mixed population of cells. Other investigators expanded the migration pattern of crest cells and determined that cells migrate in waves and give rise to specific structures along the neural axis of the embryo (Noden, 1975; Bronner-Fraser & Cohen, 1980). For example, in the 2.5-day chick embryos, melanocytes systematically migrated to the sensory ganglia, sympathetic ganglia, adrenal medulla, metanephric primordia, aortic plexus and some into the gonads (Bronner & Cohen, 1979).

Neural crest cell detachment occurs in craniocaudal waves at the anterior end of the neural tube. This population is the origin of pigmented nuclei (centers) found throughout the brain. The caudal portion of the neural crest gives rise to melanocytes and glial cells (Catala, *et al*, 2000).

Brain melanin is known as neuromelanin. When viewed in a midsagittal section of the human brain, these pigmented nuclei are strategically located around the deep cavities of the brain called ventricles as circumventricular organs (CVO). The CVO include: 1) area postrema in the fourth ventricle, 2) median eminence, 3) neurohypophysis (posterior pituitary), 4) organum vasculosum of the lamina terminalis, 5) pineal gland (epiphysis cerebri), 6) subfonical organ (SFO), 7) subcommissural organ (SCO), and 8) choroid plexus (Ganong, 2000). In other words, neuromelanin is present in neurons at sites that suggests important functions. These CVO neuromelanin have been mapped throughout the brainstem and diencephalon (Bogerts, 1981; Sapper & Petito, 1982; Cowens, 1986).

Histological studies showed that neuromelanin granules are located in the cytosol of neurons surrounded by a double membrane (Hirosawa, 1968). The brain is a highly complex organ that numerous investigators are involved in trying to understand more of its various structures and functions. It is composed of neuronal tissue, which consists of two major cell types: neurons and neuroglia. The neuron is the functional unit of the nervous system. Neuroglia (astrocytes, oligodendrocytes, microglia and ependymal cells) act as glue that fill up most of spaces between neurons as well as participate in numerous other brain functions. For example, astrocytes assist in establishing and maintaining the blood-brain-barrier. It has been estimated that there are more than ten billion neurons in the brain that receive and transmit electrical signals throughout the body. Within the soma (cell body) of a neuron are pigment granules that act like batteries that generate current for impulse transmissions away from the soma via extensions called axons; while dendrites receive input and transmit them toward the cell body.

Neurogenesis

Neurogenesis is defined as the transformation of neuroepithelial cells in committed fully differentiated nerve cells. They are determined by embryologically by two factors, sonic hedgehop (SHH) and fibroblast growth factor 8 (FGF 8) that induce the formation of dopamine producing neurons (Simon, Bhatt, et al 2003). In spite of the understanding that brain tissue is static and does not regenerate itself in adult mammalian brain, early scanning electron microscopy results show subependymal (hypendymal) cells sending out axon-like processes and subsequently migrating away from the tissue to cortical area (Privat & Leblond, 1972). Data reported by Gould, et al, (1997, 1998, 1999) show neurogenesis (new nerve and glial cell formation) in the adult primate neocortex. They reported that new neurons are added to three areas of the brain required for cognitive function: the prefrontal cortex, inferior temporal cortex, and, posterior parietal cortex. However, they appear to diminish by stress (Gould, 1998, 2001). They found no new neurons in the primary sensory area (stria cortex) involved in visual input. The subventricular area was found to contribute stem cells that migrate through the internal capsule (white matter) to the neocortex where they "sprout" new axons (new neurons). Other investigators have shown The many subcortical pigmented nuclei and their neuron circuitry contribute to the complex plasticity of the brain that begins its wiring early during embryonic development and provide new neurons throughout the life of the organism (LaCerra & Bingham, 1998).

As evidenced from recent studies using various experimental models such as mice (Synder, et al, 1997; Magavi & Macklis, 2001; Chichung, et al., 2002). A diminished population of dopaminergic neurons in the striatal pathway are said to lead to characteristics of Parkinson's disease. Additional information on neurogenesis is provided (see King, in accompanying chapter).

There seems to be species differences and age distribution variations of catecholaminergic-containing neurons, with the guinea pig and rabbit with none, and the rat, cat and dog some, higher primates more, and *Homo sapiens* highest (Mann & Yates, 1983). The differences (King, 1990) in quantity of neuromelanin may suggest that neuromelanin is not a toxic end product, or just a pigmented waste product or some detoxicating protective mechanism, but it may play a major role in electrical impulse transmission throughout the brain tissue that may be related to the flow of consciousness. It has been emphasized (Barr, 1983; Lacy, 1984), that neuromelanin has semiconductive properties such as phonon-electron coupling as in the Amorphous Theory. Simply stated, the theory says that during an action potential, neuronal phonons are transmitted through the cell and absorbed by neuromelanin granules. With changes in neuromelanin semiconduction (threshold switching), phonons are produced and transmitted via gap junctions between cells, influencing the polarization and permeability of ions via an all-or-none phenomenon (McGinness, *et al*, 1974). King (1990) states that since a great majority of catecholamine melanin-containing neurons are dopaminergic, that in general they may be involved in conscious perception, movements, emotions and memory. Comparing pigmented versus nonpigmented neurons, pigmented neurons could process information differently, or more efficiently (McGinness, 1985).

Neurotoxin MPTP and its Effect on Neuromelanin

It has been suggested that neuromelanin may play a critical role in protecting neurons from high ionizing radiation and other harmful substances such as free radicals, heavy metals, and heroin-like neurotoxic agents. Such neurotoxic agent: MPTP (1-methyl-4-phenyl-1,2,3,6-tetrahydropyridine), selectively destroys substantia nigra neurons due to the accumulation of its toxic metabolite, methylphenylpyridine (MPP+) in melanin granules of primates (D'Amato, *et al*, 1986; Lindquist, 1987; Levi, *et al*, 1989; Zecca, *et al*, 2001). When the synthetic MPTP is administered to humans or primates, they develop Parkinson-like symptoms (Barbeau,

1985). The active form, MPP+, is thought to poison the electron transport system (ETS) complex I and destroys mitochondria and selectively destroys dopamine-producing neurons of the substantia nigra (Yantiri & Anderson, 1999). These investigators suggested that iron and MPTP may work cooperatively to deleterious effects by depleting cells of free radical protections (superoxide dismutase (SOD) and glutathione peroxidase), since these enzymes were protective in transgenic and knockout mouse studies. Therefore, MPP+ accumulates via neuromelanin uptake causing toxicity and neuron cell death by inhibition to mitochondrial ATP production via NADH dehydrogenase and coenzyme Q depletion and loss of glutathione and calcium (Barbeau, 1986; Jenner, 1989). In addition, MPP+ mediates oxidative stress and neurotoxicity via the dopamine pathway, catalyzed by iron in the *substantia nigra pars compacta*. High levels of iron seen in Parkinson's patients and the neurotoxin, MPTP, can cause accumulative neurodegeneration of dopaminergic neurons, depleting the cells of neuromelanin required for impulse generation (Larsson, 1993). Iron-induced free radical formation has been implicated in Parkinson's disease (Beard, *et al*, 1993).

Neuromelanin in the Brain Cavities

The deep cavities of the cortex and its cells are discussed separately to show connections and that their lining cells contain pigmented cells. These deep cavities are part of the phylogenetic ancient brain. During embryogenesis, neuromelanin with its alternating dark and light band gaps on the UV-visible spectrum have the ability to absorb photons of light that is not re-radiated out into the system and, therefore, facilitate in the organizing deeper complex biological and developmental structures (Bynum, 1999).

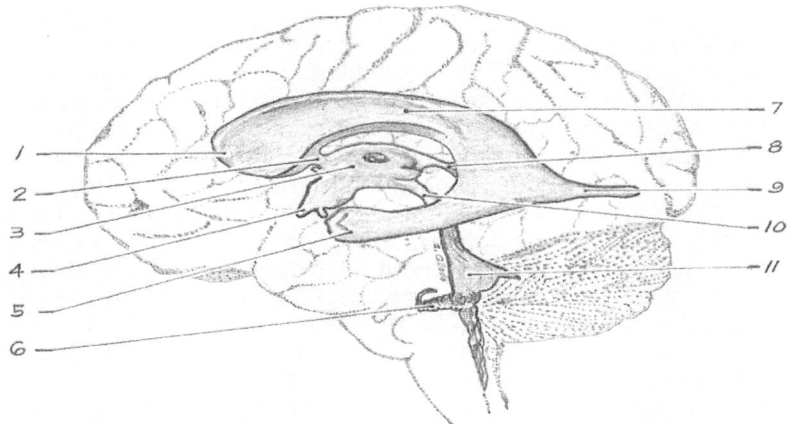

Figure 1. Cast of the Ventricles of the Brain (Lateral view).
1. Anterior horn
2. Interventricular foramen
3. Third ventricle
4. Optic recess
5. Inferior horn
6. Lateral recess
7. Body of lateral ventricle
8. Suprapineal recess
9. Posterior horn
10. Cerebral aqueduct
11. Fourth ventricle

Figure 1 is a cast of the deep cavities (ventricles) found in the cerebrum that shows the communication of the four cavities (ventricles) in the developed brain. Two ventricles are located within the cerebral hemispheres (lateral ventricles) and a third ventricle/choroid plexus in the upper brainstem of the diencephalon and a fourth ventricle/choroid plexus located between the cerebellum and the brainstem. The choroid plexus is believed to secrete most the cerebrospinal fluid. The lateral ventricles are closed cavities except where they communicate with the third ventricle via two interventricular foramina (foramina of Monro). The fourth ventricle communicates with the third ventricle of the pons and medulla through the cerebral aqueduct (aqueduct of Sylvius) of the midbrain and by three apertures (unpaired median apereture (foramen of Magendie) and two lateral apertures (foramina of Luschka) that direct the cerebrospinal fluid into the subarachnoid space. The fourth ventricle contains highly pigmented centers called the locus coeruleus (Scott, *et al*, 1973). The fourth ventricle continues caudally as a narrow central canal through the gray matter of the spinal cord. All four cavities of the ventricular system are lined with an epithelium of ependymal cells that secrete cerebrospinal fluid involved in many brain functions. Deep to the cerebral hemisphere (subcortical areas) are masses of nuclei or centers of gray matter called *basal ganglia* (caudate nucleus, putamen, globus pallidus, claustrum and amydala) that also contain neuromelanin (Akert, 1969; Smith, 1970).

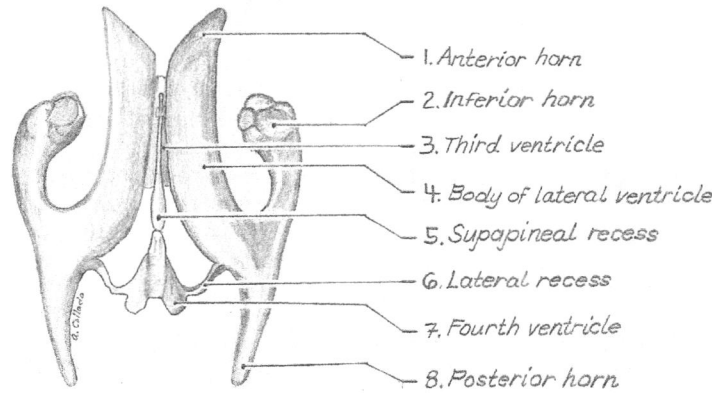

1. Anterior horn
2. Inferior horn
3. Third ventricle
4. Body of lateral ventricle
5. Supapineal recess
6. Lateral recess
7. Fourth ventricle
8. Posterior horn

Figure 2. Cast of the Ventricles of the Brain (Dorsal view).

Figure 2 is another view of these ventricular (cavities) directed for the dorsal (top) view showing their communicative connections. Cerebrospinal fluid bathes these cavities. These masses form the portion of the ventricular wall, separated by white (myelinated) fibers. Again, these pigmented nuclei have been shown to be critical in many functions such as motor (skeletal muscle) activity. Data have been presented to show that, collectively, the pigmented cells are responsible for the programming, inception and termination of motor movement. The symptoms observed in Parkinsonism are consistent with the degeneracy observed in these areas.

Biosynthesis of Neuromelanin

The steps involved in the synthesis of neuromelanin are still under debate. Some investigators argue that its synthesis is from a series of enzymatic steps similar to those established in eurmelanin (brown-black melanin) and others argue that its presence in the *substantia pars compacta* is from autoxidation of dopamine derivatives (Odh, *et al*, 1994; Zecca, *et al*, 2001, 2002). Recently, Tief and Beerman (1998) reported that melanin synthesis of proteins from extracts of adult mouse brain where they detected tyrosinase promotor gene activity in the cerebral cortex, olfactory system, hippocampus, epithalamus (pineal) and *substantia nigra pars compacta* areas that corresponded to positive staining during embryogenesis. They further stated that tyrosinase and tyrosinase-related proteins (TRP-1 and TRP-2) have been shown by others to be expressed in neural crest-derived melanocytes and retinal pigmented epithelium. They concluded that tyrosinase promotor activity is active throughout murine brain development and could be the enzymes required for neuromelanin biosynthesis. Strong evidence of the synthesis of neuromelanin by been documented by the Sulzer (2000) team.. Experimentally, they induced neuromelanin in rat ventral midbrain substantia nigra and cultured PC-12 cell line with L-DOPA   (an intermediate in the neuromelanin pathway). Using electron paramagnetic resonance (EPR), they demonstrated that L-DOPA was converted to dopamine in the cytosol and that the newly converted pigmented granules were localized in double membrane vesicles identical to that observed in the *substantia nigra pars compacta* of humans. These researchers were able to abolish neuromelanin synthesis by adenovirus constructs and concluded that neuromelanin results from excess catecholamine not in vesicles in the cytosol and subsequently stored in vesicles.

The controversy of the biosynthesis continues. Is it similar to skin melanin? Is tyrosine hydroxylase the rate-limiting enzyme in the dopamine/neuromelanin pathways, or is it tyrosinase? Whatever its origin, neuromelanin presence in critical areas of the brain/eye/ear functions is evident by its decrease in cell death seen in Parkinsonism and Alzheimer's disorder and other neurodegenerative diseases. With advances in brain research technology, instruments with strong sensitivity such as MRI and immunocytochemistry techniques, it is now possible to probe the deeper areas of the brain for clues of tissue damage and cell death. With such probe technology, is it then possible to determine if the loss of neurons manifested as degeneracy or neuromelanin loss in such neurons and other brain cells cannot function in a normal manner? Recently scientists were able to probe the memory-related structures of the brain for cellular degeneration in cases of Parkinsonism and Alzheimer's diseases (Shu & Wu, *et al*, 2002). Their findings have consistently pointed to a decrease in neuromelanin-bearing nerve cells.

Relationship of Neuromelanin in Parkinson's and Alzheimer's Disorders

One of the oldest neurodegenerative dementias observed clinically in humans is Parkinson's disease. It is associated with defective catecholaminergic neurons and neural circuitry. Specifically, there is a deficit in dopamine (neuromelanin) of the midbrain neurons. The neurotransmitter, dopamine as well as acetylcholine play a major role in skeletal muscle movement and other functions. A representative summary of this widely studied dementia by the *National Institute of Environmental Health Sciences, 1999 and Science-Week Focus Report,* make the following points: (a) The disease affects more than 1 million people in North America. That age is a consistent risk factor. (b) Parkinson's disease occurs throughout the world in all ethnic groups, mainly after 50 years of age. Its lowest prevalence is among Asians and African Blacks, and highest among Whites. (c) Clinical symptoms include tremor, rigidity, slurred speech, uncontrolled voluntary motor movements. (d) There is a progressive cell death of the dopaminergic pigmented nuclei and neural circuitry in the substantia nigra (midbrain region), as well as other subcortical pigmented nuclei that are responsive to the complex plasticity of normal brain functions. (e) The mechanisms responsible for cell death in Parkinson's disease are said to be unknown. Some of the mechanisms include genetic factors, increasing age, environmental factors, immune factors, free radical toxicity and nutrition (dietary) factors.

In some Parkinson's patients with abnormal intracellular accumulation of protein inclusions called alpha-synuclein, components of Lewy bodies have been observed in the substantia nigra (Marsden, 1983; Ballard, *et al*, 1998; Double, 1999). Treatment is based on clinical symptoms and attempts to restore some of the intermediates in the neuromelanin pathway, L-DOPA (3,4-dihydroxyphenylalanine) to be converted to dopamine, for example. Numerous labs are at work examining neuromelanin-containing neuron populations in tissue (cell) culture in the presence of L-DOPA, (Sulzer, 2000), in an attempt to understand the relationship of these neurons and their role in the disease. There is not necessarily an age limit for Parkinson's disease. For example, Pope John Paul II shows symptoms of Parkinson's disease in which his left arm shakes uncontrollably at rest, while his head tilts sharply to the right. Other Parkinson's patients that show similar symptoms include ex-boxer Mohammed Ali, Michael J. Fox, former U.S. Attorney General Janet Reno. We feel that neuromelanin plays a major role in the formation and transmission of neurotransmitter substances from one neuron to others as signals for consciousness and intellect to be facilitated.

Alzheimer's disease is the most prevalent neurodegenerative disorder in humans. It involves a loss of normal capacity to reason, think, recognize and function. This means that certain brain cells and neurons are damaged followed by cell death due to the accumulation of neurotoxins in neurons (Cafe', *et al*, 1996). Two pathologies that are hallmarks of this disorder abnormal clumps (now called amyloid plagues) and tangled bundles of fibers (presently called neurofibrillary tangles of axons and dendrites) Masliah, 2000). Again age is an important risk factor. It has been observed from imaging techniques seen in Alzheimer's patients, that there is a calculated loss of nerve cells that affects memory and language. Specifically, cell loss and cell death have been demonstrated in the hippocampus, the cortical area that deals with the storage (learning) and retrieval (memory) of information (Gage & Eriksson, 1998), while in other neurons abnormal deposits of proteins called alpha-synuclein and ubiquitin within the vesicles with Lewy bodies creates "sticky" plaques, causing the nerve axons to retract, twist, curl and coil, preventing the transport of neurotransmitter release from the axon jeopardizing nerve transmission (Sulzer, 2001). Many Alzheimer patients tend to be forgetful, especially of recent events. As the disease progresses, the patient becomes confused and may forget where they reside. Later, they may have problems speaking, reading, writing, and understanding and tend to wander away from home. The causes of Alzheimer's disease have not been fully established. Implications for nerve damage are similar to those of Parkinson's disease and may, in fact, be a different manifestation of a similar disorder, that is, a loss of neuromelanin needed for impulse formation. Again, the contributing causes are related to neurotoxins, inadequate nutrient molecules to regenerate new neurons below a critical level to effectuate electrical energy transmission for consciousness and other functions. These pathologies not only affect motor skills but behavioral functions as well (Moore, 2002).

Prevalence data shows that about 50,000 new cases (symptoms) are diagnosed in the United States each year. In 1989, this prompted the then President George Bush to sign into law the House Joint Resolution 174, declaring the 1990s as the "Decade of the Brain," making available more research funds for neuroscience research. Recent studies show that African-Americans and Asians are less likely to exhibit Parkinson symptoms than those of European descent, even though some investigators have concluded that Asians and African Blacks have a lower incidence compared to American Blacks and Whites (Lang, *et al*, 1998). In light of this discussion, the differences in prevalence of neurodegenerative diseases in the major races may be due to the neuromelanin biochemistry and nutritional intake in these cultures. There is a need to re-examine the types of food that can re-supply the cells throughout the body with those pigments found in food as raw materials for nerve regeneration and maintenance. The cost of Parkinson's disease in the United States is estimated to surpass $5.6 billion annually. The average patient spends about $2,500 annually on medication. This cost put an economic strain on the geriatric population with fixed income who are already on many other medications. Many of these patients are unable to financially manage costs that exceed their medical coverage. The African-American Parkinson's patient is less able to pay the $25,000 for the overall surgery to install electrodes needed to reduce tremors. Therefore, health care in the elderly is prohibitively costly.

The Role of Free Radicals and Free Radicals Scavengers in Parkinson's Disease

A free radical (FR) is a chemical species capable of independent existence that contains one or more unpaired electrons that occupies an atomic or molecular orbital by itself (Halliwell & Gutteridge, 1984). Such unpaired electrons cause a chemical species to be paramagnetic (attracted slightly to a magnetic field) and thus highly reactive. Free radicals are unstable due to the existence of at least one unpaired electron in its outer orbital. It is the pairing of the electrons that renders them stable. Unpaired electrons have a tendency to form a chemical reaction with another chemical species and creates a potential danger, which can cause harm to the cellular mechanisms, especially involving oxygen ions (Gerschman, 1959).

The oxygen free radicals or ROS (reactive oxygen species) include: superoxide anion, hydroxyl radicasl, lipid peroxyl radical, singlet oxygen, hydrogen peroxide and hypochlorous acid. Most the transition metals contain unpaired electrons and can qualify as radicals. This especially true with iron (Fe). Iron (Fe^{+2}) and hydrogen peroxide (H_2O_2) can react with many organic molecules such as many occur in neural tissue. This reaction has become known as the *Fenton Reaction*(Fenton, 1894). When combined, the superoxide anion and hydrogen peroxide can be scavenged in the presence of the transition metal, Fe, acting as a catalyst decreasing FRs in a combined reaction known as the *iron-catalyzed Haber-Weiss Reaction* (Haber & Weiss, 1934). The reaction is summaried as

$$O_2^- + H_2O_2 \xrightarrow{\text{Fe-salt}} O_2 + OH^- + OH^*$$

(Superoxide anion)   (Hydrogen peroxide)   (Oxygen) (Hydroxyl radical)   (Hydroxyl anion)

Cells have multiple indigenous protective mechanisms against FR damage in the form of free radical scavengers (FRS). Many of these protective molecules are classified as antioxidants. For example: Vitamin C (ascorbic acid), beta-carolene, witamin E (tocopherols), glutathione, and enzymes such as superoxide dismutase (SOD), catalase, and organic peroxidases. Experimentally, it has been demonstrated that normal cellular functions may become disturbed or altered when an abnormal balance of FRs or FRS are present in the cellular environment (Brown & Lutton, 1988; Kensler & Taffe, 1986). Glutathione has been shown to be a major FRS tripeptide found in most mammalian cells in that it facilitates the destruction of quasi-stable hydrogen peroxide and other organic peroxides, when can generate toxic FR species (Kuthman & Eriksson, 1979). The Glutathione Cycle used by the cell the scavenge FR species plays a critical role in the detoxification of ROS (Brown, 2003, minireview).

The major function of FRS, glutathione, is to protect the cell against endogenous FRs and other oxygen stressors. In neurodegenerative diseases such as Parkinsonism as well as Alzheimer's diseases, FR are thought to be produced within the deep cerebral nuclei called basal nuclei and can lead to progressive damage and nigral death. (Zeevalk, Bernard & Ehrhart, 2003).   Recent evidence suggests that membrane lipids in the substantia nigra show typical signs of oxidative damage, suggesting FR injury via lipid peroxidation (incorporation of ROS in the membrane lipid moiety of neuronal cells) (Hirsch, 1993; Jenner & Olanow, 1996; Simonian & Coyle, 1996; Sudha, Rao & Rao, 2003). Studies of glutathione (GSH) depletionin in vitro and in vivo in the presence of the neurotoxin, MPTP, increased ROS in mice suggesting potential damage to midbrain neurons (Sriram, Pai, K.S., *et al*, 1997).

     The debate continues as the exact etiology of neurological disorders in patients with Parkinson's and Alzheimer's diseases. It is theoretical possible that oxidative stress can occur in neuronal tissue because of an imbalance in the FR/FRS production and the ability of the neurons in the brain to protect and prevent these cytotoxic radical formation, leading to a progressive , long-term deterioration of motor functions.

     Although, a scarcity of scientific research is available on the role of nutrition as an underlying cause of neurodegenerative disorders, poor nutrition habits over many years may contribute to many brain disorders. For example, high consumption of meats and metal toxicity metabolically can generate ROS that can damage normal tissue, especially when antioxidant glutathione and other free radical scavengers are reduced. A daily intake of foods such as of fruits, vegetables, nuts and seeds (especially when consumed raw) contribute molecules that are supportive good health and wellness. Nutrition is an area that needs to be thoroughly examined and documented. Poor nutrition of many may be one of the main contributing causes of Parkinson's and Alzheimer's diseases. In addition, there is some hint that years of negative thinking such as *fear,* resentment, worry, bitterness, anger, as well as body toxic load may have a strong effect on the overall health. Nerve cells are certainly influence by the biochemical milieu from the blood stream.

Natural Plant Pigments in Foods are Required for Normal Nerve Functions

    At the beginning of this work, the ubiquity of black material in the universe was well documented. Investigators have shown the presence and importance of this dark pigment (melanin/neuromelanin) in the cytoplasm in trillions of nerve cells in the brain. It was advanced that neuromelanin is concentrated in neurons in strategic areas of the brain that is key to maintaining the flow of impulses throughout the brain continuously that we call *consciousness.* This very powerful matter acts as low level semiconductors (superconductors), transmitting and regenerating the current needed for consciousness, intellect, sensory and motor functions. It is our position that neuromelanin is regenerated through raw food and food pigments intake, especially from raw fruits and vegetables and natural unprocessed food additives.

Much attention has been focused on Alzheimer's disease, an insidious neurodegenerative brain disorder that results in memory loss, unusual behavior, and regressive thinking ability. These neurological patterns are said to be related to the death and destruction of brain nerve cells ,connective tissue and supporting cells called neurolgia. The preceding sections describes neuromelanin deficiency of Alzheimer's and Parkinson's brain disorders. This section advances the notion that oxygen, natural (not synthetic) food pigments can prevent the coagulation of toxic protein in the nerve cell body and neurofibrillary abnormal twisting that results in memory loss due to the inability of nerve impulses to be propagated (review-UCLA Alzheimer's Disease Research Center).

For more than three decades scientists have thoroughly documented the protective effect of one natural food ingredient curcumin, a yellow, pigmented chemical constituent derived from tumeric and other spices used in foods (Lin, et al 1994).

Over 100 Western studies, and still growing, and many more by Indian scientists, have already demonstrated that natural plant-derived phytochemical, polyphenolic pigments in common foods additives ingested daily in cultures such as Indian (Ayurvedic), African, Carrebean, Asian and South American, can prevent orreduce many of the neurological and other debilitating diseases seen in Western cultures where these additives are rarely used. In particular, studies show that low doses of Curcumin (Curcuma longa), a yellow, active ingredient in curry and tumeric, may reduce or prevent conditions ranging from Alzheimer's to certain viral diseases (Aggarwal, Kumar and Bharti, 2003). This would suggest that food pigments are biochemical molecules that are as important as vitamins, minerals and other foods components and must be included in the daily consumption of foods for healthy nerve functioning.

Studies done on the elderly Indian opoulation that has regularily consumed large amounts of tumeric spice in their diet was likely to develop Alzheimer's or multiple sclerosis (MS) than their counterparts in the Western population (Natarajan and Bright,2002). In view of this, Western scientists theorized that curcumin, a component in temeric spice, must contain anti-inflammatory properties. This finding was supported by a finding that Westerners taking anti-inflammatories regularily for arthritis are less likely to develop Alzheimer's disease (Halliday, Robinson and Kril, 2000).

Recent studies theorizes that curcumin may effectively cross the blood-brain barrier and bind to toxic beta amyloid proteins in the brain of Alzheimer's patients and break up existing plaques and prevent the formation of others (Yang et al, 2004). Furthermore, curcumin has powerful anti-oxidative and anti-inflammatory properties in low doses that ease disease symptoms causes by oxidation and inflammation (Huang et al.,2004 ; Kelawata and Ananthanarayan, 2004; Yang,2004; Frautschy,2001),chemoprotective in the growth of gastric and colin cancer (Mahady et al. 2002) and may protect the brain against free radical damage by the induction of heme oxygenase as protection (Scapagnini, et al.,2004).

It is our position that a great deal of the pain and suffering visited upon the world's elderly population especially, are nutrician related. In spite of food distribution injustices there are other advantages that poor countries have that run circles around more affluent countries in their cultural selection of foods that tend to keep certain disease states at a minimum.

We further hypothesize that pigment-bearing raw food substances makes available biochemical molecules used by nerve cells to regenerate its neuromelanin that the cell bodies of millions of neurons require moment-by-moment semiconductors (superconductors) and propagation of impulses that we call consciousness. Any obstruction of this current flow by foreign toxic matter such as toxins from years of a waste in the colon and re-circulated to the brain, ties binds to the neuromelanin and may be contributing factors to Alzheimer's pathology seen in hippocampus brain tissue or rigidity and tremors due to lack of neurons and its neuromelanin in the midbrain in Parkinson's disease. It is the author's observation that at the site of a synapse, there is neuromelanin that receives and recharges the impulse. A second look at neuromelanin as semiconductor in neurons needs to be carefully examined to find answers to age-old brain disorders. More on nutrician in disease etiology is forthcoming in a separate work.

Conclusion

Melanin is a biopolymeric pigment with semiconductor properties. It is present within the cells of all living things. Since these pigments are present from the beginning of inception, these bioactive pigments play a major role in the cellular/molecular and embryological organization of all living things. Neuromelanin is present in neural tissue and appears to function in the transduction and flow of electrical current from one part of the brain to another through a complex circuitry. In brain tissue, data shows that neuromelanin located within dopaminergic and adrenergic neurons may exhibit properties that qualifies it as both a biological superconductor and as an amorphous semiconductor— a threshold switch, similar to that of inorganic materials (McGinness, *et al*, 1974 and post-publication not 2001). This post-publication note says that: *"melanins give a flash of light when they switch–clearly electroluminescence, though its significance is not completely understood at this time."* Does this flash contribute to what is called spirituality, the ability to utilize the brain energy for consciousness and healing qualities? In the brain, could this flash of light generated by such amorphous semiconductivity between low to high threshold switching of neuromelanin be analogous to "consciousness?" If this is the case, then this neural dark matter also is the light that makes it possible to "see." And, if neuromelanin pigment is stored within vesicles, its synthesis may be required as a continuous source of current whose product is the neurotransmitter substance. Some of these ideas need to be discussed and, where possible, investigated from a new perspective to gain additional answers to health issues.

In the context of health related research we have also note that natural pigments found in foods and spices are beneficial to the regeneration of neuromelanin found in the body, especially in the brain where the pigment is key as a semiconductor that propagates electrical currents continuously via trillions of neurons that allows consciousness and other functions to give life. Elderly persons in cultures where spices such as tumeric (curcumin) is a regular food additive rarely suffer debilitating diseases such as arthritis, Alzheimer's and certain other neurodegenerative diseases. Tumeric (curcumin) has anti-oxidative, anti-inflammatory and cytoprotective peoperties by acting as a scavenger of reactive oxygen species that may contribute to the formation of beta-amyloid plaques, which sequesters neuronal cytoplasmic neuromelanin and other toxic chemicals, causing some of the symptoms seen in the nervous system.

In addition, the neuromelanin of the neuronal-neuroglia ventricular system may activate and then transmit consciousness to all parts of the brain for cognition and motor activity. Data clearly shows that a decrease in midbrain dopamine-bearing neuron/neuroglia population results in a loss of the functions of motor activity, speech, learning, and memory as seen clinically in Parkinson's and Alzheimer's disorders (Kastner, et al, 1992). In some patients, the axons and dendrites of neurons in certain areas of the brain are twisted and coiled, preventing neurotransmitter flow from one nerve to another, which contributes to pathologies and cell death. The specific causes of these neurodegenerative disorders has not been clearly established. There appear to be multifactorial factors such as genetic inheritance, the environment, increasing age, free radical toxicity, neurotoxins, and nutrition. Drugs exert cumulative negative effects, especially in people of color, that contribute to behavioral modifications. The importance of these effects needs to be taught to our children, especially nutritional contributions. Yes, dark matters (Moore, 1995, 2002) and our scientific perspective should be expanded and explored to include an African-centered perspective. Nevertheless, there is some hope in addressing some of these disease symptoms observed in areas of the brain such as the hippocampus and the basal ganglia (dentate gyrus) of adult monkeys that lean towards stem cell that "sprout" into new neurons to replace damaged cells (Gould, et al, 1997,. 1998, 1999, 2002). Finally, we would encourage some open, honest scholarly discussions be given to the meaning of this neural dark matter as it relates to behavior, emotions, learning, intelligence, health, well-being, aging, and longevity in non-pathological conditions.

References

Aggarwal,B.B.,Kumar,A. and Bharti,A.C. (2003) Anticancer potential of curcumin: preclinical and clinical studies. *Anticancer Res.*23 (1A), 368-98.

Akbar, N.(1984). *Chains and images of psychological slavery.* Jersey City, NJ: New Mind Productions.

Akert, K. (1969). The mammalian subfornical organs. *J. Neuro Visceral Rel. (Suppl. IX)* 78- 93.

Ballard, C., Grace, J. & Holmes, C.(1998). Neuroleptic sensitivity in dementia with Lewy bodies and Alzheimer's disease. *Lancet* 351, 1032-1033.

Barbeau, A. (1985). Comparative behavioral biochemical and pigmentary effects of MPTP, MPP+ and paraquat in *Rana pipiens. Life Sci.*37, 1529-1538.

Barbeau, A. (1986). Environmental and genetic factors in the etiology of Parkinson's disease. *Adv. Neurol.* 45, 299-306.

Barnes, C. (1988). Melanin: The Chemical Key to Black Greatness, Vol. 1. Black Greatness Series, Houston, TX, pp. 56, 57.

Barr, F. (1983). "Melanin: The organizing molecule". In: *Medical Hypotheses* 11, 1-140.Review

Beard, J.L., Connor, J.D. & Jones, B.C.(1993). Brain iron: location and function. *Prog. Food Nutr Sci* 17, 183-221. Review.

Bogerts, B. (1981). A brainstem atlas of catecholaminergic neurons in man, using melanin as natural marker. *J. Comp. Neurol.*197, 63-80.

Bonner, M.E. & Cohen, A.M.(1979). Migratory patterns of cloned neural crest melanocytes injected into host chicken embryos. *Proc. Natl. Acad. Sci. U S.A.* 76, 1843-1847.

Bonner Fraser, M. & Cohen, A.M.(1980). The neural crest: what can it tell us about cell migration and determination? *Curr. Top. Dev. Biol.* 15 Pt 1,1-25. Rev.

Bynum, E.B. (1999). The African Unconscious. Roots of Ancient Mysticism and Modern Psychology. Teachers College Press, p. 100f.

Brown, A.C. (2003). Glutathione: Free Radical Scavenger That Protects Against Cell Damage, *In Vivo* 24(1), 4-10.

Brown, A.C. and Lutton, J.D. (1988).The significance of free radicals and free radical scavengers. *Advances in Experimental Medicine and Biology* 241, 135-148.

Café, C., Torri, C., Bertorelli, L. et al.(1996). Oxidative stress after acute and chronic application of beta amyloid fragments 25-35 in cortical cultures. *Neuroscience Lett.* 203,61- 65.

Chichung, Lie, D., G. Dziewczapolski, A.R., Willhopite, et al. 2002. The adult substantia nigra contains progenitor cells with neurogenic potential. *J. Neurosci.* 22,6639-6649.

Catala, M., Ziller, C., et al.(2000). The developmental potentials of the caudalmost part of the neural crest are restricted to melanocytes and glia. *Mech. Dev.* 95, 77- 87.

Cohen, A.M. & Konigsberg, LR. (1975).A clonal approach to the problem of neural crest determination. *Dev Biol.* 46, 262-280.

Cope, F. W. (1978).Discontinuous magnetic field effects (Barkhausen noise) in nucleic acids as evidence for room temperature organic superconductors. *Physiological Chemistry and Physics, 10, 233-245.*

Cope, F. W. (1981). Organic superconductive phenomena at room temperature. Some magnetic properties of dyes and graphite interpreted as manifestations of viscous magnetic flux lattices and small superconductive regions. *Physiological Chemistry and Physics, 13, 99-110.*

Cotzias, G.C., et al.(1964).Melanogenesis and extrapyramidal diseases. *Fed. Proc.* 23,713-718.

Cowens, D.(1986). The melanosomes in the human cerebellum (nucleus pigmentosis cerebellaris) and homogules in the monkey. *J. Neuropath. Exper. Neurol.* 45, 205-221.

D'Amato, R.J., Lipman, Z.P., & Snyder, S.H. (1986). Selectivity of the parkinsonian neurotoxin MPTP: toxic metabolite MPP+ binds to neuromelanin. *Science* 231,987-989.

Diop, A.C. (1991). *Civilization or barbarism: An authentic anthropology.* Brooklyn, NY: Lawrence Hill Books.

Double, K.L., Riederer, P., & Gerlach, M.(1999). Significance of neuromelanin for neurodegeneration in Parkinson's disease. *Drug News & Perspectives*, 12, 6.

Double, K.L., Zecca, L., et al.(2000). Structural characteristics of human substantia nigra neuromelanin and synthetic dopamine melanins. *J. Neurochem.* 75,2583-2589.

Frautschy,S.A., Hu,W.,Kim,P. et al. (2001) Phenolic anti-inflammatory antioxidant reversal of A3-induced cognitive deficits and neuropathology. *Neurobiology of Aging* 22(6),993-1005.

Gage, F. & Eriksson, P. (1998). Neurogenesis in the adult human hippocampus. *Nature Med.*4,1313- 1317.

Ganong, W.F. (2000). Circumventricular organs: definition and role in the regulation of endocrine and autonomic function. *Clin. Pharmacol. Physiol.* 27,422-427.

Gerschman, R. (1959).Oxygen effects in biological systems.*Proc. Int. Congr. Physiol. Sci.* 21st Buenos Aires,pp.222-226.

Gould, E., et al. (1997). Neurogenesis in the dentate gyrus of the adult tree shrew is regulated by psychosocial stress
 and NMDA receptor activation. *J. Neurosci.*l7, 2492- 2498.

Gould, E., Tanapat, E., McEwen, B.S., et al. (1998). Proliferation of granule cell precursors in the dentate gyrus in adult monkeys is diminished by stress. *Proc. Natl. Acad. Sci. U.S.A.* 95, 31689-31710.

Gould, E., Beylin, A., Tenapat, P, et al. (1999). Learning enhances adult neurogenesis in the hippocampal formation.*Nature Neurosci* 2,260-265.

Gould, E., Vail, N., Wagers, M. & Gross, C.G.(2001). Adult generated hippocampal and neocortical neurons in macaques have a transient existence. *Proc. Natl. Acad. Sci.U.S.A.* 98,10910-10917.

Gould, E. & Gross, C.G. (2002). Neurogenesis in adult mammals: some progress and problems. *J.Neurosci.*22,619-623.

Graham, D. G.(1978).Oxidative pathways for catecholamines in the genesis of neuromelanin and cytotoxic quinones. *Mol.Pharmacol.*14,633-643.

Halliday,G.,Robinson,S.R.,Shapherd,C., and Kril,J., (2000).Alzheimer's disease and inflammation: a review of cellular and theraputic mechanisms. *Clin. Exp. Pharacol. Physiol.* 27(1-2),1-8.

Halliwell, B & Gutteridge, J.M.C. (1984).Oxygen toxicity, oxygen radicals, transition metals and disease. *Biochem. J.* 219, 1-4.

Harsa-King, M.(1980). Melanogenesis in oocytes of wild type and mutant albino axolotls. *Dev. Biol.* 74, 251-262.

Hendrie, H., Ogunniyi, A., Hall, K.S., et al. (2001). African Americans develop Alzheimer's disease and other dementias at twice the rate of Africans. *JAMA* 285,739-747.

Hirsch, E.C. (1993). Does oxidative stress participate in nerve cell death in Parkinson's disease. *Neurology* 33 (suppl 1), 52-59.

Hirosawa, K. (1968). Electron microscopic studies on pigment granules in the substantia nigra and locus coeruleus of the Japanese monkey (*Macaca fascularis yakui*). *Z. Zellforsch Anat* 88, 187- 203.

Huang, X.,Moir, R.D.,Tanzi,R.E.,Bush,A.L., and Rogers,J.T. (2004). Redox-active metals, oxidative stress and Alzheimer's disease pathology. *Ann N.Y. Acad. Sci.*1012. 153-163.

James, G.M. (1954). *Stolen Legacy*. New York: Philosophical Library, United Brothers Communication Systems.

Jenner, P. (1989). Clues to the mechanism underlying dopamine cell death in Parkinson's disease. *J. Neurol. Neurosurg. & Psychiatry* 22,28.

Jenner, P. and Olanow, C.W. (1996). Oxidative stress and the pathogenesis of Parkinson's disease. *Neurology* 47 (suppl 3),S161-S170.

Kastner, A., Hirsch, E.C., *et al*. (1992). Is the vulnerability of neurons in the substantia nigra of patients with Parkinson's disease related to their neuromelanin content? *Neurochem.* 59,1080-1089.

Kelawata, N.S. and Anathanarayan,L. (2002).Antioxidant activity of selected foodstuffs.*Internat.J.Food Science and Nutrician* 55,511-516.

King, R.D. (1990). Selected References to the Eye of Heru from Pyramid Texts, Durham, North Carolina.

King, R.D. (1994). The African Origin of Biological Psychiatry. U.B. and U.S. Communications, 912 Pembroke, Hampton, Virginia 23669.

King, R. (2001). Melanin: A Key to Freedom. Lushena Books, Inc. 1804 West Irving Park Road, Chicago, IL. 773-975-994.

Kozlowsky, G.P., Scott, D.E., & Dudley, G.K. (1973).Scanning electron microscopy of the third ventricle in sheep. *Z. Zellforsche* 136, 169-176.

Lacy, M.E. (1984). Phonon electron coupling as a possible transducing mechanism in bioelectronic processes involving neuromelanin. *J. theor. Biol*.111,201-204.

LaCerra, P. & Bingham, R.(1998). The adaptive nature of the human neurocognitive architecture. An alternative model. *Proc. Natl. Acad. Sci. U.S.A.* 95, 11290-11293.

Lang, A.E & Lozano, A.M. (1998). Medical Progress: Parkinson's disease. Parts 1 & 2. *New England Journal of Medicine*, 339, 1130-1143:1040-1053.

Larsson, B.S. (1993). Interaction between chemicals and melanin. *Pigment Cell Res*.6,127-133.

Levi, A.C., DeMattei, M., *et al.* 1989). Effects of 1- methyl-4-phenyl-1,2,3,6-tetrahydropyridine (MPTP) on ultrastructure of nigral neuromelanin in *Macaca fascicularis*. *Neurosci. Lett*. 96,271-276.

Lim, G.P., Chu,T., Yang.F.,Beech.W.,Frautschy,S.A., and Cole,G.M., (2001) The curry spice curcumin reduces oxidative damage and amyloid pathology in an alzheimer's transgenic mouse. *J.Neuroscience* 21(21),8370-7.

Lin,J.K., et al (1994).Molecular mechanism of action of curcumin,in :**Food Phytochemicals II: Teas, Spices, and Herbs**. *American Chemical Society*,20,196-203.

Lindquist, N. G. (1987).Neuromelanin and its possible protective and destructive properties. *Pigment Cell Res*. 1, 133-136.

Mahady, G.B.,Pendland,S.L., Yun,G.,and Lu,Z.Z.(2002). Tumeric (*Curcuma longa*) and curcumin inhibit the growth of *Helicobacter pylori*, a group 1 carcinogen. *Anticancer Res*. 22(6C),4179-81.

McGinness, J., Corry, P. & Proctor, P. (1974). Amorphous semiconductor switching in melanins. *Science* 183, 853-855.

McGinness, J.(1985).A new view of pigmented neurons. *J.theor.Biol*. 115,475-476.

Magavi, S.S. & Macklis, J.D. (2001). Manipulation of neural precursors in situ: induction of neurogenesis in the neocortex of adult mice. Neuropsychopharmacology 25, 816-835.

Mann, D.M. & Yates, P.O. (1983). Possible role of neuromelanin in the pathogenesis of Parkinson's disease. *Mech.Age Dev.* 21,193-203.

Marsden, C. D. (1983). Neuromelanin and Parkinson's disease. *J. Neural Transm. Suppl. 19*,121-141.

Mason, H. S. "Structure of melanins " In: *Pigment Cell Biology* (Myron Gordon, ed.). Academic Press, Inc. Pub., New York, 1959, p.581.

Masliah, E. *et al.* (2000). Dopaminergic loss and inclusion body formation in alpha synuclein mice: implications for neurodegenerative disorders. *Science* 287,1265-1269.

Moore, T. O.(1995).The Science of Melanin. Dispelling the Myths. Venture Books/Beecham House Pub. Inc.

Moore, T. O.(2002). Dark Matters Dark Secrets. Zaman Press, Redman, Georgia.

Natarajan,C. and Bright,J., (2002). Curcumin may block progression of multiple sclerosis. Annual Experimental Biology 2002 Conference, New Orleans, LA (April 23,2002).

National Institute of Environmental Health Sciences NIEHS Fact Sheet Parkinson's Disease Research, April 1999.
http://www.niehs.nih.gov/ and http:www.scienceweek.com.

Nicholaus, R.A. (1997). *Coloured organic semiconductors: melanins.* Rend. Acc. Sci. Fis. Mat.,LXIV, 325-340.

Nicholas, R. A., Patel, M. & Fattorusso,E.(1964).The structure of melanins and melanogenesis IV. *Tetrahedron* 20,1163.

Nicholas, R. A. & Piattelli, M. (1965). Progress in the chemistry of natural black pigments. *Rend. Acad. Sci. Fis. Mat.*, Naples, 32, 83-97.

Noden, D.,(1975). An analysis of the migratory behavior of avian cephalic neural crest cells. *Devel. Biol.*, 42, 106-130.

Odh, G., Carstam, R., *et al.* (1994). Neuromelanin of the human substantia nigra: a mixed type melanin. *J. Neurochem*. 62,2030-2036.

Ono, K., Hasegawa,K.,Naiki,H. and Yamada,M. (2002). Curcumin has potent anti-amyloidogenic effects for Alzheimer's beta-amyloid fibrils *in vitro. J. Neuroscience Res*. 75(6), 742-50.

Pavan, W.J. & Tilghman, S.M.(1994). Piebald lethal (sl) acts early to disrupt the development of neural
crest derived melanocytes. *Proc. Natl. Acad. Sci. U.S.A.* 91, 7159-7163.

Privat, A. & Leblond, C.P.(1972). The subependymal layer and neighboring region in the brain of young rat. *J.Comp. Neurobiol.*146, 277-301.

Robinson, K.P. (1979). Electrical currents through full grown and maturing Xenopus oocytes. *Proc. Natl. Acad. Sci. U.S.A.* 76, 837 841.

Rugh, R. (1977). A Guide to Vertebrate Development, (7`h Ed.) Macmillan Pub. Co., NY, p 56.

Sapper, C.B. & Petito, C.K.(1982). Correspondence of melanin pigmented neurons in human brain with Al-A14 catecholamine cell groups. *Brain* 105,87-101.

Scapagnini, G. Colombrita, C.Calabrese,C., Pascal,A., Schwartzman,M.L. and Abraham,N.G. (2004). Curcumin cytoprotective effect in rat astrocytes and neurons is mediated by specific induction of HO-1, presented at *Experimental Biology 2003 Conference*, Washington, D.C., April 17-21, 2004.

Schraermeyer, U. (1996). The intracellular origin of the melanosome in pigment cells: a review of ultrastructure data. *Histol. Histopathol*. 11,445-462.(A review).

Scott, D.E., Kozlowski, G.P., *et al.* (1973). Scanning electron microscopy of to human cerebral ventricular system. II. The fourth ventricle. Z. Zellforschung 139 64 68.

Shu, S.Y., Wu, Y.M., Bao, X.M., *et al.* (2002). A new area in the human brain associated with learning and memory: immunohistochemical and functional MRI analysis. *Mol. Psychiatry* 7,1018-1022.

Simonm H.H., Bhatt, L.,Gherbassi, D.,Sgado,P.,and Alberi,L.(2003). Midbrain Dopaminergic Neurons. Determination of Their Developmental Fate by Transcription Facrs. *Ann. N.Y. Acad. Sci.* 991,36-47.

Simonian, N.A. & Coyle, J.T.(1996). Oxidative stress in neurodegenerative diseases. *Annu. Rev. Pharmaco.l Toxicol.* 36,83-106.

Smith,U.(1970).Aspects of the fine structure and function of the subcommissural organ of the embryonic chick. *Tissue & Cell* 2,19-32.

Spemann, H. (1938). Embryonic Development and Induction. Ch. VIII. Yale University Press,New Haven, Connecticut. 401pp.

Sriram, K.,Pai, K.S., Boyd, M.R.& Ravindranath,V.(1997).Evidence for generation of oxidative stress in brain by MPTP: in vitro and in vivo studies in mice.*Brain Res.*749(1),44-52.

Synder, E.Y.,Yoon, C, Flax,J.D.& Macklis,J.D.(1997). Multipotent neural precursors can differentiate toward replacement of neurons undergoing targeted apoptotic degeneration in adult mouse neocortex. *Proc. Natl. Acad. Sci.* USA.94,11663-11668.

Strzelecka, T.(1992).A band model for synthetic DOPA melanin. *Physiol. Chem. Phys.* 14,219-233.

Sudkha, K, Rao, A., Rao,S.,Rao,A.(2003).Free radical toxicity and antioxidants in Parkinson's disease. *Neurology India* 51 (1),60-62.

Sulzer, D., Bogulavsky, J., *et al* (9 authors). (2000). Neuromelanin biosynthesis is driven by excess cytosolic catecholamines not accumulated by synaptic vesicles. *Proc.* Natl. *Acad. Sci. U.S.A.* 97, 11869-11874.

Swart, H.M.,Sarna, T.& Zecca, L.(1992). Modulation by neuromelanin of the availability and reactivity of metal ions. *Ann. Neurol. 32* (Supply, S69 S75).

Tief, K., Schmidt, A. & Beermann, F. (1998). New evidence for presence of tyrosinase in substantia nigra, forebrain and midbrain. *Brain Res. Mol. Brain Res.* 53,307-310.

Weston, J.A.(1982).Neural crest cell development. *Prog. Clin. Biol. Res.* 85(Pt B), 359-379.

Yang,T.,Lim,G.P.,et al.(2004). Curcumin inhibits formation of A-b-oligomers and fibrils and binds plaques and reduces amyloid *in vitro. J. Biol. Chem.*, 10,1074 (on line).

Yantiri, F. & Andersen, J.K. (1999). The role of iron in Parkinson disease and 1-methyl-4-phenyl-1,2,3,6-tetrahydropyridine toxicity. I(JBMB *Life* 48,139-141.

Zecca, L., Macacci, S., Seraglia, R.,& Parati,E.(1992). The chemical characterisation of melanin contained in the substantia nigra of human brain. *Biochim. Biophys. Acta* 1138,6-10.

Zecca, L., Tampellini, D., Gerlach,M.,*et al.*(2001).Substantia nigra neuromelanin: structure, synthesis, and molecular behavior. Mol. Pathol. 54,414-418.

Zeevalk, G.D., Bernard, L.P. & Ehrhart, J. (2003).Glutathione and Ascorbate. Their Role in Protein Glutathione Mixed Disulfide Formation during Oxidative Stress and Potential Relevance to Parkinson's Disease, *Ann. N.Y. Acad.Sci.* 991,342-345.

CHAPTER 3

The Clinical Use of Bliss: A Standardized Technique For Conscious Intervention into the Functioning of the Autonomic Nervous System (ANS)

by

Edward Bruce Bynum, Ph.D., ABPP.[1]

"All animals have an internal core of melanin in their brains. All humans possess this Black internal brain evidence of their common Black African origin. The all black neuromelanin nerve tract of the brain is profound proof that the human race is a Black race, with many variations of black, from Black-Black to White-Black.... One of the critical keys that distinguishes man from all other animals is this presence of intense blackness, neuromelanin pigmentation of the locus coeruleus, Black Dot, the upper most center of pigmentation, the doorway that opens into an all black hall of blackness, the neuromelanin "Amenta" nerve tract."

Address all correspondence to Edward Bruce Bynum, Ph.D.,ABPP, Director of Behavioral Medicine, University of Massachusetts Health Services, 127 Hills North, Amherst, MA 01003 USA

The author is indebted to the following people for their technical comments and expertise in the review of this paper:

T. Owens Moore, Ph.D., Professor of Psychology, Clark Atlanta University and the Neuroscience Institute Morehouse School of Medicine;

Alan J. Calhoun, M.D., Medical Director, University of Massachusetts Health Services;

Warren H. Morgan, M.D. Associate Medical Director, University of Massachusetts Health Services.

Richard D. King, M.D.
African Origin Of Biological Psychiatry

> "Brain melanin (neuromelanin) increases with ascent up the phylogenetic ladder, reaching a peak concentration in man. Moreover, it is invariably found in strategic highly functional loci of the brain... Neuromelanin within neurons and glia is concentrated in strategic locations of the brainstem which (together with monoaminergic axonal and dendrite extensions) allow for the " gating" of all sensory and motor input and output as well as all emotional and motivational input and output."

F.E. Barr, M.D.
Melanin: The Organizing Molecule

> A standardized clinical technique for conscious and directive intervention into autonomic nervous system functions is presented along with a description of both subjective and psycho physiological reactions to this technique. Its use with numerous symptoms and conditions is discussed as a means to decrease stress producing somatic dysfunctions and increased focused relaxation of psycho physiological processes. Potential pathways and underlying mechanisms of the technique and operations are also discussed as it relates to the midbrain limbic system and the somatic unconscious. The process of physiognomic perception is discussed. The role of neuromelanin in somatic and other nervous system operations is elaborated.

KEY WORDS: Kemetic, neuromelanin, melanin, autonomic nervous system, limbic system, alternate nostril breathing, meditation, hemispheric dominance, physiognomic perception, acupuncture, nadis, psycho physiological equipoise, locus coeruleus, biological superconductivity, quantum resonance, Dogon of Mali.

Overview and Statement of the Problem

In many different clinical fields a skilled intervention into autonomic nervous system functioning is crucial for therapeutic work. This is true whether working in the field of behavioral medicine, in biofeedback specifically, or in the related field of clinical hypnosis. In each one of these fields the autonomic nervous system is often a focus for intervention since often its delicate balancing operation is seen to underlie the manifestation of somatic symptomatology. With so many diverse procedures and practitioners in these clinical fields, there is a need for a standardized technique for conscious and skilled intervention with the autonomic nervous system. This technique or procedure would need to be capable of selectively influencing the autonomic nervous system. In addition to that the technique should be demonstrated to the patient with only minimal regard for experimental and experimenter bias. It is a technique that should be able to be taught in a *standardized* way in order to elicit *standardized responses* from the patient. It is also preferable that it be a technique that can affect the autonomic nervous system while the patient is fully conscious and in control of their psychological and physical faculties. What follows therefore is a brief article on a clinical technique that is in operation in specific therapeutic settings focused within a certain constellation of somatic symptoms. It will also offer the psycho physiological and psychological concomitants and repercussions of this technique. We will then discuss how this technique can be used with various clinical situations. Finally this chapter will propose some ideas as to why this technique is clinically effective. We will also discuss the psychological and psycho physiological basis for the efficacy of the technique and its relationship to other disciplines in the alteration and transformation of consciousness.

Brief History

The history of therapy and healing has always been intimately associated with the clinical practitioners' capacity to affect the autonomic nervous system and human consciousness. Any successful therapeutic methodology had to offer an explanation to the patient or sufferer as to the how and why of their predicament. The explanation needed to be consistent with the worldview of the time and era of the therapeutic setting.

In each setting it was and is the clinical and ethical task of the clinician to listen closely to the patient, communicate verbally and nonverbally that someone with training and education cares about them, that the patient's symptoms are explainable in some way and that their symptoms and condition are controllable or at least amenable to therapeutic influence. This communication allows the clinician a conscious entrance into both the patient's unconscious and autonomic system, and also what we would term the patient's interpenetrating bio-informational energy field.

The clinical settings of today often use " scientific " modern metaphors such as computer analogies, conscious/unconscious dichotomies, and other "modern language" to describe what is actually an ancient discovery. (Bandler and Grinder, 1982;Bandler and Grinder, 1981; Hourning, 1986) Even in ancient Kemetic Egyptian times and then in later Greek and Roman times, the intervention into the autonomic nervous system using various procedures such as clinical hypnosis, auto-suggestion and other techniques to decrease or eliminate the numerous stress-related "dis-eases" and pain syndromes was well testified to in the classical literature. (Muses, 1972;Edmonston, 1986;Ebbell, 1937) Due in large measure to the practice of mummification the original indigenous Emetic Egyptian knowledge of anatomy and physiology was quite extensive and precise, only to be surpassed 3 millennia later in the 18th century in Europe (Finch 1990). Much as their practices laid the foundation and template of human civilization (Diop, 1974; Jackson, 1970), their developing practices and knowledge of the body essentially became the template of Western scientific medicine. With the advance of modern anatomy, neuroanatomy and psychophysiology however, we have been able to progressively and more clearly delineate exactly the psycho physiological processes that are involved in these procedures. Clearly many of the ancient cultures had sophisticated methods for the treatment of a wide variety of symptoms, symptoms we still see in clinical practice today. (Finch, 1990) The technique that we are going to be elaborating here draws from many different sources, but in particular modern psychophysiology, neuroanatomy, certain Yoga practices, an awareness of specific acupuncture correspondences and some forms of a higher cortical skill or "emergent mental disciplines" known as meditation. In concert these disciplines can exercise a controlling influence on lower order symptom phenomena operating in the body-mind. Given, as earlier chapters have pointed out, the intimate interplay between melanin, neuromelanin, bioelectrical conductivity and the central nervous system, the operation of consciousness and neuromelanin will become more pronounced as this chapter unfolds.

Description of the Technique

The technique itself falls into three phases. We will elaborate the psycho physiological basis of each of those phases as this article progresses. At the present time it should be noted that the three phases are comprised of: (1) diaphragmatic breathing; (2) alternate nostril breathing; and (3) a particular focus of attention on a specific area of the body and then the " re-awakening" of this sensation in clinically focused regions of the body. These, when done in sequence, provide a replicatiable demonstration of specific stimulation of the autonomic nervous system under the direct control of the person's attention and focus.

The first phase involves diaphragmatic breathing. This means directly teaching the patient by demonstration on oneself to differentiate between chest or thoracic breathing and diaphragmatic breathing. In the process of doing this the patient will experience an observable and undeniable sensation. The clinician can then draw the patient's attention to certain psycho physiological processes that are stimulated by diaphragmatic breathing. After the diaphragmatic breathing occurs for approximately 5 to 8 minutes the patient is then taught alternate nostril breathing. Alternate nostril breathing, a well-established Yogic technique that affects the ANS, serves to deepen and intensify the psycho-physiological reactivity that has already been initiated by the diaphragmatic breathing. (Kuvalayanandal, 1978; Funderbunk, 1977;Thakkur, 1977) The alternate nostril breathing is usually done at a slow pace anywhere from 3-5 minutes. Then, after alternate nostril breathing has followed the procedure of diaphragmatic breathing, the patient is taught to relax and focus their attention at a place on the top of the lip and bottom of nose. The patient's attention is drawn subtly to the alternating current of slightly warm then cool then warm air again they can notice at the top of the lip, bottom of nose area. . When this three-part pattern is done *in sequence* the patient has a definite observable psychophysical response that the clinician can then draw the patient's attention to. It leads to a decidedly "blissful" feeling and sometimes to the actual organismic perception of a "blissful current" coursing through the body along a certain pathway. This blissful sensation in its clearest form is a non-ideational, somewhat luminous sensation not identified with any specific organ or site but one that may, when directed, pervade that region. It has an affinity to the sensation that occurs immediately anterior to a strong sexual orgasm and also to the somatic memory of the body and mind in deep sleep without dreaming where there is little or no thought but certainly an intuition of bodily and psychological restoration and rejuvenation. We will have more to say about this later in this paper. This whole procedure takes approximately 10 to 12 minutes to do successfully. After that point the patient's attention is then drawn clinically to whatever *areas* of the body-mind are the focus for clinical intervention.

What follows next is a two-part description of the psycho physiological and the psychological experience of the patient executing this procedure. First the subjective experience is presented.

Subjective and Somatic Experience of the Procedure

The procedure initiates a number of clearly observable subjective experiences on the part of the patient. The patient initially feels more "relaxed." In some patients there is an initial paradoxical response of increased anxiety before relaxation. However in the majority of patients relaxation is the first noticeable sign. With continual practice the patient begins to notice that there is a gradual slowing down in their subjective perception of the "speed" of their thoughts. Also the patient often spontaneously begins to notice more imagery emerge from their experience. Sometimes this imagery is associated with immediate experiences, sometimes long forgotten memories come to the surface again. The unconscious is accessed by this procedure.

In terms of their psychophysiological experience, a number of things become noticeable during the procedure. A large percentage of patients witness during this phase an increase in saliva in the mouth. There is also an increase in heat on the surface of the skin due to vascular dilatation, and an increase in GI tract activity in a pleasant direction as though one were getting ready for a meal. The patient may also spontaneously notice that certain areas of the body, particularly the clinically effected areas of the body, become more clear in terms of their visualization and organismic perception of this area. Finally a significant number of patients will notice a "tingling sensation" all over the surface of the body, in particular around the face and the limbs. These occur in varying degrees. The clinician, while observing the patient, can observe some of these processes and selectively amplify or reinforce them for clinical effect. With this increase in psychophysical reactivity, shifts in somatic perception and subjective experiences of relaxation and even euphoria and blissful sensations at times, the patient can begin to notice the capacity for potentially altering sensory experience. (Erickson and Rossi, 1979) Patients are engaged in this immediate experience and also, in conjunction with biofeedback equipment, can gain direct biomedical information concerning their symptoms and psychophysical reactions by way of proprioceptive feedback from certain areas of the body.

For instance a patient can notice an increase in heat in localized regions of the body or generalized all over the surface of the body. This is due to increased blood flow or vascular dilatation. This is useful when certain symptoms involving circulatory or cardiovascular problems are the target of clinical focus, e.g. common and classical migraine headaches, labile high blood pressure, dysmemorrhea, Raynaud's disease, Berger's Disease, and other related phenomenon. There is also a decided increase in the feeling of identification with and subjective relaxation in certain areas of the body. This is due to the relaxation of specific muscle groups. This is a useful technique in dealing with issues involving muscular and motoric constriction and/or spasticity, e.g. GI tract disturbances (IBS etc), muscle contraction headache, chronic pain syndromes, etc. However, the procedure is not limited to these systems alone. Others, such as the respiratory system, are affected, making it possible to treat asthma, rhinitis and related symptomatology. A number of clinical studies have indicated that an increase in relaxation and a decrease in psychophysical reactivity and decrease in stress chemistry lead to an increase in immune-enhancement or immune functions. (Locke and Colligan, 1986; Kiecolt-Glaser et al, 1985; Achterberg and Lawlis, 1984; Rider et al, 1990) It is well known that harmful stress hormones are decreased by calm imagery and thought, that painkilling endorphins and the immune system can be modulated by therapeutically guided mental states. There is enormous potential for the patient. This technique allows the patient, with progressively deepening skill and "emergent" higher order cortical control processes, to interact consciously and specifically, with the soma and therein to literally "talk" to certain areas of the body. By teaching the patient a skillful observational method and a way to intervene in this psycho physiological process of the body, the patient learns to selectively enhance or decrease the reactivity of certain somatic functions. In this process the patient spontaneously remembers or associates in an affectively charged way to certain images, ideas and motifs that can be clinically quite useful in a psychotherapeutic context. The psychological and somatic regions of the unconscious are accessed. There is a certain affinity here between clinical hypnosis, imagery and autosuggestion. In the context of biofeedback, however, these can be enhanced significantly and accurately due to the nature of the psycho physiological monitoring feedback process.

It is very important to note at this juncture that the surface of all these internal organs along with the entire surface of the brain, crucial regions of the mid-brain, parts of the endocrine system, autonomic nervous system and the peripheral nervous system all have significant amounts of this semi-conducting melanin and neuromelanin in them as part of their structure and content. It is suggested here that in ways we are only now beginning to understand this complex and interwoven bioinformational field generated in early embryogenesis and developing throughout the life cycle communicates with itself via conductivity and sometimes, under the right conditions, consciousness.

Psychophysiological Description of the Procedure

What follows next is a closer and clearer description of each one of the three sequential stages of the technique. Each one will be presented in more detail along with its psycho-physiological basis.

The first phase of the procedure is referred to as diaphragmatic breathing. Diaphragmatic breathing, as opposed to chest or thoracic breathing, involves the movement of the abdomen and the diaphragm in the breathing process. (Fried, 1987) Breathing air into the deep recesses of the lungs is almost always a healthy activity. The pericardium is attached to the diaphragm and thus the process of deep breathing causes the diaphragm to descend, stretching the heart slightly downward toward the abdomen. When the lungs are filled with air from the bottom upwards, they compress the blood rich viscera, giving a gentle massage to the heart and the internal organs. As the diaphragm then contracts and releases, it also massages the heart, pancreas, liver, stomach, small intestine, abdomen and other internal organs. This leads to a better diffusion of blood through the system and a gentle stimulation of the internal organs. (Lysebeth, 1983; Rama, Ballentine and Hymes, 1979) This internal process affects the autonomic nervous system with observable results.

The human nervous system can be divided structurally into the central and peripheral branches. The peripheral branch is subdivided functionally into the somatic branch, which is generally conscious, and the involuntary or autonomic branch, which is generally unconscious. The autonomic nervous system itself is subdivided into two branches, the sympathetic and the parasympathetic nervous system branches. See Chart #1.

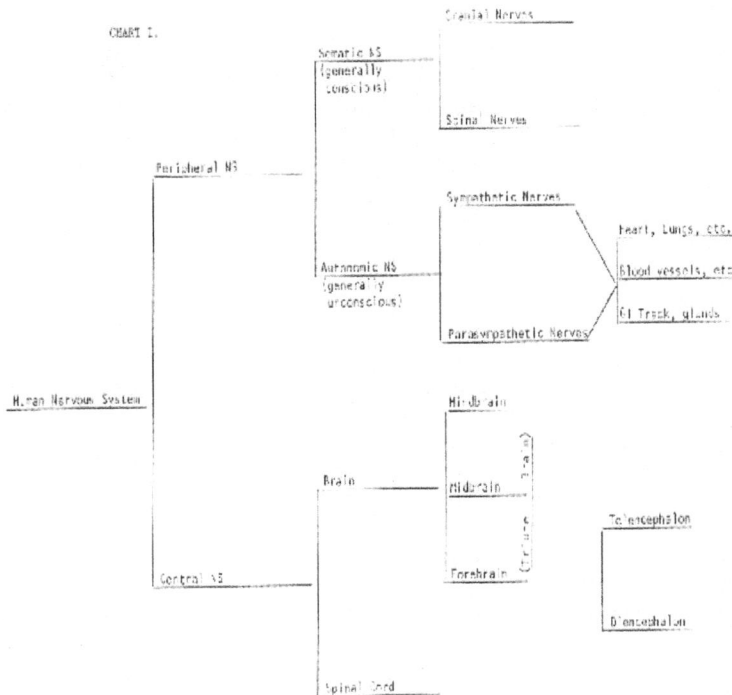

These branches usually work in balanced opposition with each other such that there is an overall harmonious regulation as the net result. For example, in cardiac functions the parasympathetic system focuses on slowing down the heart rate while the sympathetic system is involved in increasing the speed of the heart rate. Their dynamic balance is the ideal for lowered levels of stress. Symptoms often arise when there is a sustained imbalance in either one. In the case of accelerated heart rate, (tachycardia), or slowed heart rate, (bradycardia), arrhythmias of several kinds may eventually arise resulting in a variety of well known clinical syndromes. Psychological stress and/or depression can lead toward certain arrhythmias, innumerable psychosomatic disorders or to the suppression of immunocompetence systems. (Locke and Colligan, 1986;Achterberg and Lawlis, 1984) See Chart #2.

The sympathetic nervous system consists mainly of two vertical rows of ganglia or constellations of nerve cells arranged on both sides of the spinal column. Their branches spread out to all of the different organs, glands and internal systems of the abdomen, thorax and other areas of the body. They also intermingle in integrated plexuses with nerve branches of the parasympathetic system. It is significant that a principal part of this system is the tenth cranial nerve also called the vagus or the wandering nerve. It is connected to the hindbrain and travels downward along the spinal cord through the neck, chest, abdomen and other vital organs sending out its branches into various nerve constellations with the sympathetic system. It ends in a constellation, which is connected to the solar plexus. However even though it may end in the solar plexus, it still sends thin filaments to lower levels of the body. (Netter, 1972; Tokay, 1972) In clinical practice when the patient begins to slowly and methodically regulate the motion of the lungs, the heart itself is slowly regulated. Eventually the right vagus nerve is brought under conscious control and thereby that area of the brain that is implicated in the involuntary or autonomic systems of the body is made amenable to *conscious influence* on the part of the patient. (Rama, Ballentine and Hymes, 1979)

To the extent that the mind becomes focused it then is capable of extending or amplifying this capacity to volitionally influence the body. The metaphor of a laser that focuses the diffuse light of the mind or consciousness into a coherent light that is then capable of a different kind of work is often used with the client to demonstrate this principle. From this vantage point there is no area of the body-mind that is not in some degree amenable to conscious influence by the higher cortical centers of the brain and consciousness. Eventually, in the process, the patient's attention is progressively drawn more and more into the *exhalation* phase of the breathing cycle. This gentle emphasis on the exhalation phase of the breathing cycle differentially reinforces the parasympathetic branch of the autonomic nervous system leading to a decrease in conventional stress for most of the organ systems. (Rama, Ballentine and Hymes, 1979)

The autonomic nervous system has a complicated series of interactions and innervations with the different organ systems of the body. As a general rule, the sympathetic system creates tension and constriction in the systems and the parasympathetic system creates relaxation or dilatation. There are a few exceptions to this generalization. The pupils of the eye and the bronchi of the lungs initiated by intense interest or anxiety are examples of the opposite of these tendencies. See Chart #1.

After the patient has mastered diaphragmatic breathing their attention is then drawn to alternate nostril breathing. It is of interest that the nasal passages have a cycle of approximately 1 1/2 to 1 3/4 hours of dominance of one nostril (Klein and Armitage, 1979). In other words, for approximately an hour and a half to an hour and forty-five minutes the left or right nostril is more dominant allowing air to pass more freely through its turbinates. The nasal system is actually a neurological system in that the first cranial nerve, the olfactory or the one that we smell with, has subtle nerve endings in the top of the mouth, bottom of the nose. These olfactory cells are presently the only known sensory cells to conduct impulses. These olfactory cells originate in the nasal mucosa. They course through the cribriform plate to the olfactory bulb, then backward and along the olfactory nerve below the frontal lobe dividing into two branches. It is unclear whether the medial branch in humans ends in the subcallosal gyrus and the parolfactory area. The lateral branch does terminate in the uncus and, very importantly, in the emotional and "meaningful" memory processing hippocampus gyrus (Netter, 1972).

It is curious and clinically significant that each time we inhale and exhale we stimulate this nerve and this sends a subtle message to the midbrain limbic system, the system that supervenes over our primitive emotionality, e.g. flight-fight response, disgust, gustatory, etc. Furthermore this midbrain limbic system consisting of the amygdala, hippocampus and hypothalamus, is deeply implicated in the generation and filtering of powerful unconscious emotions ranging from lust to rage, to murderous impulses to spiritual intoxication and anomalous experiences that alter our perception of space, time, location and reality (Joseph, 2000). Many primitive emotions and reactions and their coordinated bodily functions from respiration to cardiac functions to gastrointestinal motility are stimulated in this way. This is why we look to the limbic structures for the root of this bodily current of primal feeling. It is essentially our "emotional body".

When the tenth cranial nerve or vagus nerve in particular is stimulated by way of this deep diaphragmatic breathing with an emphasis on the exhalation phase of the breathing cycle the hormone epinephrine that arises in the body *outside* these neural structures and the neuromodulator norepinephrine that arises *within* these neural structures are brought into interaction(Hassert, Miyashita and Williams,2004). This release of norepinephrine quickly floods the amygdala thereby stimulating and deepening the memory of powerful positive or negative emotions and experiences from the "emotional body". Because the hormone epinephrine cannot cross the blood-brain barrier that enfolds these mid-brain structures the ascending or afferent fibers of the vagus nerve that pick up the stress chemistry produced by the adrenal medulla in the flight-fight response in turn stimulates the neurons in the brainstem known as the nucleus of the solitary tract (Hassert, Miyashita and Willams, 2004).From there the message is then transmitted to the ancient mid-brain limbic system for "meaningful" consolidation by both the amygdala and perhaps the hippocampus.

These mid-brain limbic structures that communicate feeling and emotion then can flow, interface with bodily sensations and "project" to other areas of the brain. The motor projections from the spinal line up are to the anterior or pre-central gyrus and the sensory projections are to the post central gyrus. Both gyri have the body topologically outlined on the surface. There are innumerable connections by nerve fibers of varying degrees of myelination and by long pyramidal tracks that twist and turn through complex and curving convolutional "spaces" before they reach their final destination in the projection areas of the cerebral cortex. It is truly awesome to see how these interweaving nonlinear spaces and fibers have woven together the different regions, spaces and functions of the cerebral universe.

Powerful emotions and feelings have been deeply rooted in the hominid neurobiological structures for millions of years. Archaic humans had religious impulses, buried their dead and experienced the full spectrum from awe to terror. Before the emergence of complex thought, speech and linguistic patterns, they had created tools, survival skills, made strong emotional attachments, and lived through lust, passion and dreams. These are rooted in the temporal lobes and midbrain limbic system. Only later as Homo Sapiens evolved toward Homo Sapiens Sapiens, our species, did there develop the capacity for initiative, long term goal setting and cognitive reflection on multiple options in any given situation. The frontal lobes have increased by %33 in Homo Sapiens Sapiens, while the limbic structures have remained essentially unchanged (Joseph, 2000). The deep core emotions of embodiment are an evolutionary neurobiological unfoldment of these limbic structures. What we outline here is a conscious way to intervene into this system.

By careful diaphragmatic breathing and alternate nostril breathing, the patient gives, by way of the first cranial nerve and the tenth cranial nerves of the somatic nervous system, a specific and soothing message to the autonomic nervous system. There is an direct experiential sense of a kind of bio-conductivity of energy and affect through the system. The net result is continual vascular dilatation, increased heat on the surface of the body, continual blood diffusion through the body, more efficient use of the lungs, and massage of the internal organs. The net effect is a more positive and consistent and "embracing" proprioceptive feedback to the body. This significantly decreases the stress reaction and the harmful effects of constant stress chemistry to one's psychophysiology. As dreams were the " royal road " to the unconscious in early psychoanalysis, conscious and disciplined respiration is the velvet path into this "somatic unconscious". Both reflect and are implicated in powerful emotional processing that occurs in the limbic and paralimbic systems of the brain.

Many experimenters have come to notice that the nasal cycle opens a certain "window" on the autonomic nervous system and an opportunity for cerebral hemispheric influence to occur. Researchers have noticed that there is a direct relationship of cerebral hemispheric activity as monitored by an electroencephalogram (EEG), and the ultradian rhythm of the nasal cycle. (Werntz, 1981) Essentially, the relatively greater integrated EEG values in one hemisphere are positively correlated with the predominate airflow in the contra lateral or opposite nostril. (Werntz, 1981; Werntz et al, 1981) Researchers have also noticed that by changing nasal dominance by the technique of forced single nostril breathing through the nondominant closed nostril that effects can be found on the EEG. Thereby *one can experimentally shift the nasal dominance and this is accompanied by a shift in cerebral hemisphere dominance to the contra lateral hemisphere*. This has been known clinically for the last decade. However, it has also been the testimonial of certain meditative disciplines, in particular the Swara yogis (Prakashan, 1980), for thousand of years. (Werntz et al, 1981) This phenomenon, clinically speaking, eventually allows for the patient to be able to voluntarily change the relative focus of activity in the higher cortical centers of the brain and thereby influence the all pervasive and supervenient autonomic nervous system reactions that regulate practically every major function of the body. By the technique of alternate nostril breathing the patient is able to differentially affect the right or left hemisphere of the brain and its associated cognitive activities.

There is some controversy as to the psychophysical basis for this reactivity. However, most researchers believe that this technique represents an extensive integration of autonomic and cerebral cortical activity. (Klein and Armitage, 1979;) It is held that the nasal cycle is itself regulated centrally by the hypothalamus, thus altering the sympathetic/parasympathetic balance. This reaction occurs throughout the body, including the brain, and is perhaps the mechanism by which all basal motor tone regulates the control of blood flow through the cerebral vessels thereby itself altering cerebral hemispheric activity. This clearly is an influence consciously of hemispheric laterality and also the limbic system upon the body by the higher cortical centers of the brain. The revolution in cognitive psychology has now established that subtle higher cortical processes can act as causal constructs in brain behavior and that indeed these mental states and skills as *emergent properties* of neurological activity definitely exercise a supervenient influence over lower order biological and psychological events. (Sperry, 1988) Regulating the system, quieting external noise or distractions and intensifying internal concentration or attention accomplish the specific influence that is exercised by this procedure. Attention to external events and stimuli is simultaneously decreased. With this done systematically, various areas of the system are brought consciously under more and more influence and control of consciousness. Thereby symptoms can be affected quite specifically.

The third phase of the procedure involves the focusing of attention on the top of the lip, bottom of the nose. The focusing here is done usually on the *exhalation* phase of the breathing cycle. The patient is often asked to lick the top of the lip with their tongue, creating a little moisture such that the alternating current of warm, then cool, then warm air again, can be noticed. After that, progressively more attention is drawn toward the exhalation phase of the breathing cycle. This area is chosen for two distinct reasons. The more overt reason is that the air current can be directly experienced here with relatively little effort. The second reason is that it tends to steady attention. But there is another reason for focusing here.

In acupuncture theory, there is a major meridian that terminates at the area of the top of lip, bottom of nose referred to as the "governor vessel meridian". (Motoyama, 1981) By focusing attention in this area, this subtle acupuncture meridian is technically activated and what is called the "chi" or "ki" energy is then moved more systematically like a river through the twelve ordinary meridians of the system. The principle underlies much of well-tested and centuries old acupuncture theory and practice. (Huang Ti, 1966) This procedure also tends to steady attention and allow a pleasurable, even "blissful current" of non-ideational feeling and sensation to arise and organismicly be perceived to move along the body axis of the spine. It tends to decrease any dominance of the sympathetic or the parasympathetic system and brings them more into a dynamic balance. Finally it should be noted that in some Yogic meditative disciplines this procedure, which follows alternate nostril breathing, helps "depotentiate" the dominate tendency of the right or the left side of the body and to allow for an opening of what is termed the "central canal." (Motoyama, 1981; Rama, 1981) There is the belief in Yoga practice that the right and left sides of the body along the spine have a conduit for the movement of energy called the Ida and Pingala Nadis. They correspond, it seems, to the second lines of the urinary bladder meridian of acupuncture. When depotentiated, the current moves into this central canal, the body axis along which a pleasant, blissful current of sensation is organismically perceived to move. The dominance of either the "right side" sympathetic nervous system innervations or of the "left side" parasympathetic system innervations is not conducive to deeper meditative states.

When the three procedures are sequentially followed and the final procedure is accomplished, it is very often useful to have the patient then begin to focus their sense of internal relaxation and psychophysical equipoise on the affected organ. When this is done, the eyes are slightly opened and internally focused on this area, or closed but still focused on this area and an inner part of the body. This procedure is very similar to the meditative procedure of Shambhavi mudra. (Svatmarama, 1971)

Subjectively this is a very powerful procedure and clinically will differentially activate or "awaken" certain areas of the body, both "subtle" and gross.

It is important to note that some patients occasionally slip into the deeper regions of this practice and experience phenomena encountered by practitioners of other associated cognitive and contemplative disciplines. In particular when the heart rate is slowed enough and coordinated with respiration, the heart-aorta system tends to produce an oscillation of about 7 hertz (Hz) that then reverberates throughout the entire skeletal framework, especially in the dense structures of the skull. This in turn is believed to create a series of standing waves projected to the ventricles of the brain stimulating the perception of a moving sensory current that flows through the entire body but which is actually focused in the neural structures. These standing waves are in multiples of the 7Hz base heart-aorta oscillation (Sannella, 1987;Bentov,1977). Other wider environmental entrainment effects have also been observed. This experience can be both intensely pleasurable but also disorienting and so should be avoided unless the patient is also practicing a specific contemplative discipline that is aware of these phenomena. The boundary between phenomena that is internal and external to the patient or practitioner also tends to become more blurred and porous and thereby the perception of inner life, activity and consciousness is easily perceived or recognized as existing throughout one's external space. "Space" itself tends to undergo various alterations at "times", an interesting area that we will return to in later parts of this chapter.

The successful execution of this procedure in a primarily clinical context however gradually brings more of the unconscious areas of the body into conscious availability and thus amelioration by biofeedback and behavioral medicine procedures. A number of clinical problems are thereby amenable to treatment. These include not only the symptoms associated with cardiovascular activities, e.g. angina pectoris, arrhythmias, migraines, elevated blood pressure, etc., and with muscular activities, e.g. TMJ, bruxism, muscle contraction headache, ulcerative colitis, IBS, etc., but also potentially those of "soft" neurological and immuniological significance (See chart II).

Chart II.

Partial List of Stress Modulated
Diseases and Symptoms

I. Cardiovascular Diseases
- A. Cardiac Arrhythmias
- B. Cerebral Stroke
- C. Anginas Pectoris
- D. Coronary Artery Disease
- E. Hypertension
- F. Raynaud's Disease
- G. Migraine Headaches

II. Muscle-Related Symptoms
- A. Tension Headaches
- B. Oral Conditions
    1. Bruxism
    2. TMJ
    3. Clenching
    4. Myofacial Pain Syndrome
    5. Necrotizing Ulcerative Gingivitis
    6. Apthous and Herpetic Lesions
- C. Shoulder Aches (Chronic)
- D. Backaches
- E. Neck aches

III. Gastrointestinal
- A. Colitis
    1. Ulcerative (Inflammatory)
    2. Spastic or Mucous
- B. Peptic Ulcer
- C. Fecal Incontinence

IV. Genitourinary
- A. Impotence
    1. Primary

        2.   Secondary
- B. Dysmenorrhea and Amenorrhea
- C. Dyspareunia and Vaginismus
- D. Eneuresis and Encopresis

V. Allergic Diseases
- A. Asthma
- B. Chronic Urticaria (Hives)
- C. Angioneurotic Edema (Allergic Swelling)
- D. Vasomotor Rhinitis

VI. Infectious Diseases (Through stimulation of the immune system).

VII. Hyperthyroidism

VIII. Rheumatoid Arthritis

IX. Diabetes Mellitus (Through disordered metabolism and hyperglycemic disregulation).

X. Cancer(s) (By way of immune system compromises).

XI. Psychological-Psychiatric
- A. Depression
- B. Insomnia(s)
- C. Anxiety Reactions
- D. Behavioral Dysfunctions, Tics, etc.
- E. Phobias

XII. Miscellaneous Diseases
- A. Neurodermatitis (Skin rash)
- B. Alopecia (Hair Loss)
- C. Graying hair (Prematurely)
- D. Hypoglycemia
- E. Thrombophlebitis

<u>Discussion and Implications: The Somatic Unconscious</u>

What follow next are some preliminary ideas on the potential neuroanatomical pathways and psycho physiological activity that may accompany the aforementioned technique. We have already mentioned the psycho physiological reactions that occur when one is practicing this procedure. Psycho physiological activity is associated with the sequence of diaphragmatic breathing, alternate nostril breathing, and the focus of attention at top of lip, bottom of nose. It is suggested that the emergent higher cortical functions of the human nervous system in this context exerts a decided influence on lower order cognitive and psychophysical activity. (Sperry, 1988) See graph # 1, a sagittal section of the human brain from cerebral cortex to cerebellum including limbic system structures.

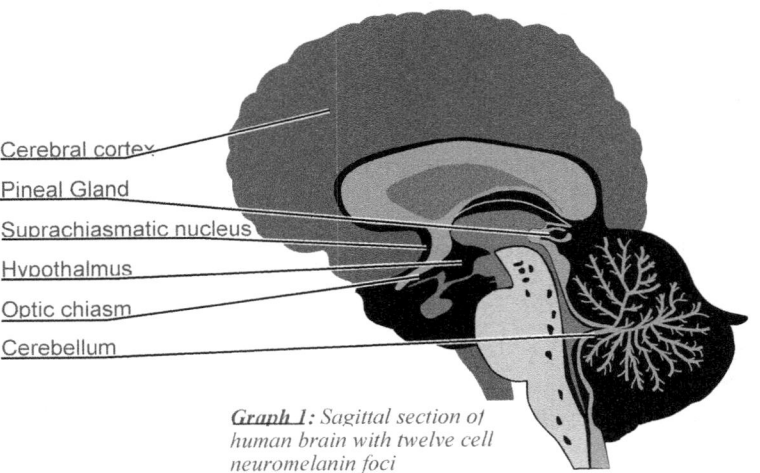

Graph 1: Sagittal section of human brain with twelve cell neuromelanin foci

In particular, the human nervous system harnessing the process of physical "tension" and psychological "attention" is able to differentially affect the peripheral and the central nervous system. A form of bio-conductivity of energy and affect is directly experienced. *The strategic locations within the brain and the sensory and motor "gateway functions" of neuromelanin(Barr,1983) in these cerebral structures identifies neuromelanin as the most likey facilitator for this activity*. In reference to the peripheral nervous system, it is generally divided into the somatic and the autonomic nervous system. See Chart #1. The somatic nervous system itself gives rise to the twelve cranial nerves and the thirty-one pairs of spinal nerves. The autonomic nervous system however, a system that is generally unconscious, is involved with the sympathetic and the parasympathetic nervous system. The sympathetic and the parasympathetic nervous systems innervates all of the central organs of the body, including the heart, lungs, blood vessels, GI tract, etc. By learning how to differentially increase or decrease stimulation to these areas using imagery and the control of respiration and attention, the first cranial or olfactory nerve to the midbrain limbic system and the tenth cranial or vagus nerve is stimulated and thereby a certain psychophysical reactivity is affected.

In terms of psychiatric symptomatology, it is notable that a specific cerebral area of the central nervous system, in particular the locus coeruleus, seems to account for approximately 70% of all central nervous system noradrenergic activity. King (1990) and others have pointed out that neuroanatomicaly the locus coeruleus occupies the uppermost point in an all black neuromelanin nerve track that runs from the brain stem into the spinal cord. It has been observed that higher levels of locus coeruleus activity are correlated with hyper vigilance and attention to unusual or fear provoking stimuli, but also less activation appears to be associated with behavior such as sleep, grooming and feeding. (Foote, Bloom and Aston-Jones, 1983) This would suggest that the locus coeruleus, an area highly associated with neuromelanin activity in the brain, acts as a controlling gate to stimuli coming into the system. In other words the signal-to-noise ratio of incoming stimuli is significantly affected by the operation of the locus coeruleus. It appears to have a rather substantial afferent input from the internal organs and seems to receive direct innervations from the medullar nucleus solitarus (Elama,Svensson, and Thoren,1986; Charney, Heninger and Breier, 1984). The medullar nucleus solitarus is an area known to be a principal locus for afferent information from the internal organs. Emotional modulation of this area due to stress, familial dynamics or other stimuli, and the perception of this area by the conscious mind, produces the emotions of anxiety, fear and potentially depression. Anxiety, depression, and fear can lead to hypo motility while aggressive feelings such as hostility and resentment can cause hyper motility (Gillis, Quest, Pagani et al, 1991). Such psychological disorders that involve anxiety and somatization may be reflected in gastro-intestinal and chronic pain syndromes. Studies have suggested that there is a pathological disregulation of the locus coeruleus in panic disorder (Gorman, Liebowitz, Fyer et al, 1989) and possibly in depression. (Charney, Heninger and Breier, 1984; Charney and Heninger, 1986; Siever, Uhde, Jimerson et al, 1984) Essentially then the locus coeruleus, an area associated with high levels of neuromelanin activity, is a possible central nervous system area having both afferent and efferent connections to the internal organs and can provide a pathway for some of the neuroactivity of the system. This locus coeruleus may combine not only internal or visceral stimuli but also midbrain limbic and higher cortical stimuli and then integrate and redistribute the information to other systems, all usually occurring outside of conscious awareness. These are midbrain limbic system expressions of what is termed the somatic unconscious. See graph # 2 of primary limbic system structures.

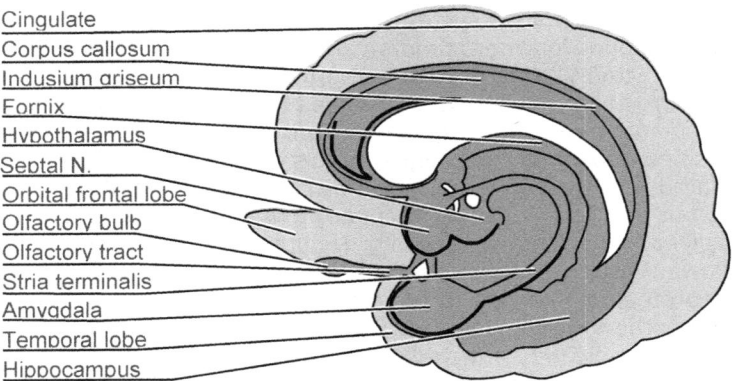

Graph 2: Limbic system primary structures

The locus coeruleus is a term of ancient lineage, deriving from the Latin word for "locus" meaning point or dot, and the Sanskrit " caeruleus yamas" meaning black (King, 1900) This "black dot" area of the brain holds a significant amount of melanin (Amaral and Sinnamon, 1977). Its cells project to and provide for the primary noradrenergic nerve supply to many other sites in the brain, including the forebrain and the cerebral cortex, but also down to the hippocampus, the cingulate gyrus, and the amygdala areas, which comprise the major portion of the limbic cortex. This locus coeruleus is also known to supply part of the norepinephrine located in other brain sites, especially the hypothalamus, the thalamus, the habenula or deep pineal, the cerebellum-lower brainstem and then the spinal cord.

We mentioned above that neuromelanin appears to play a modulating role in this system. (Moore, 1995;Moore, 2002,). It is already known that neuromelanin in all likelihood plays a high role in the modulation of catecholaminergic transmission. (Kagan and Rosenberg, 1987) The genetic or biological hypothesis presents itself here, since neuromelanin is an integral aspect from the very earliest phase of human embryological development beginning with precursors of the neural crest system itself and appears to exercise an organizing influence in this process. (Barr,1983) It is by no means conclusive but it is certainly suggestive[2].

Actually the deep brain core runs down and out the brain stem down to near the base of the spine. The spinal cord itself is an extension of that original embryonic neural crest. The spine is a longish white cylinder, oval in cross section. The inner matter is dark gray and the outer surface is white. In the brain itself this situation is reversed and the outer surface is gray while the inner bulk is white. Modern neuroscientists have shown that this light interacting melanin that creates the gray color of the brain is present in the brain of all animals with the degree of its pigmentation clearly increasing as creatures move up the evolutionary path (Marsden,1961; Scherer,1939). Mammals have the greatest density; primates have the highest among the mammals (Bogerts, 1981). Finally, even among the primates the higher the evolutionary form of brain complexity and organization or similarity to the human type, the richer the light interacting melanin and biochemistry of the brain.

---

[2] **Developmental embryology reveals that only days after conception the zygote or embryo begins to emerge eventually dividing into 3 distinct cell layers: the inner or endoderm, the middle or mesoderm and the outer or ectoderm. Each layer gives rise to specific organ systems. This unfoldment is guided by the activity of light sensitive melanin's melanocyte functioning all of which begins prior to the first heartbeat !. The ectoderm especially leads to the formation of the neural crest, the nervous and endocrine systems, the spinal line, and the epidermis. Melanin appears to be a crucial organizing molecule orienting the organism toward light from the earliest stages of embryogenesis.**

We also know that melanin itself is highly concentrated not only on the surface of the brain and crucially in specific regions within the brain core, but also, clinically speaking, on the surface of many internal organs of the viscera, the diffuse neuroendocrine system, and the sensory systems of the eye and auditory system. All of which communicate with each other in interconnected organismic pathways. This suggests a certain kind of energy and bio-informational field capable of self-regulation and conscious influence under certain conditions. This interpenetrating field responds to various forms of stimuli, in particular the potentially guiding stimuli of light, heat, sound, movement and resonance. After all melanin does absorb a rather wide spectrum of electromagnetic radiation and other energies of excitation from adjacent molecular structures. All this mind you while shielded from the ultraviolet radiation of the sun by almost half an inch of skin and skull. Clearly the brain, through the process of melanin, is absorbing radiation in both its local aspects and perhaps even partakes in its nonlocal dynamics.

Consciousness, it seems, enters or projects into this three dimensional picture through its luminous, vibratory affinity with the dynamics of neuromelanin. In other words, at the level of neurodynamics in the behavior not of the cells, but at the synaptic junctures, quantum mechanical processes seem to occur. These processes reflect the so called "state vector" collapse of nonlocal light from its all pervasive vibratory "source" into localized actuality from the vast realm of many potential states existing in multiple or "N" dimensional space. This collapse of the nonlocal may even have an affinity for the localization of forms and "shapes" in space. In a very real sense just as we might say that "matter" arises when the background "field strength" of the pure field becomes intense enough, so does the light of self-aware consciousness arise from the dark background field consciousness when its density or strength is sufficiently strong enough.The presence of darkness in neuromelanin appears to be crucial here in that both the pre-synaptic and the post-synaptic neural structures have " dense projections of gray" between which energy flows at the synaptic junctures. Whether this energy is in the form of electron tunneling or quantum "resonance" of some kind is an open question.

Our own intuition here supports a rhythmic and harmonic resonance process. Regardless of whatever model of "energy" and information transfer you perceive, the "quantum sea of Light energy" that is both matter-energy and the very potential itself of matter-energy that pervades the universe, is actualized here from the boundless background reality that gives rise to space, time, matter and all their interpenetrating, multidimensional dynamics. This is a vibratory universe, " as above, so below", and so the warm dark matter of the brain in its affinity for shapes, forms and processes must surely reflect in some way the patterns in the unseen cold dark matter of this universe. After all the brain is a product and therefore in some ways a reflection of the structures of the universe and so it is reasonable to locate some of these subtle structures and processes of the cosmos with its innumerable convolutions and interconnections of space, time and distances in the structures and processes of the brain.

Melanin and neuromelanin again have established bioelectrical[3] conductivity properties and may, under these restricted conditions manifest the phenomenon of biological superconductivity.

In this context research has established that the various midbrain limbic system structures, e.g., amygdala, hippocampus and inferior temporal lobe, are implicated in the stimulation/modulation of our primary emotions ranging from rage to love to spiritual intoxication (Joseph, 2000). The neocortical surfaces of both the amygdala and the inferior temporal lobe have "dense neural fields" that recognize and respond to geometrical shapes and emotional imagery. These neurons are often called" feature detectors". This is both in response to external and internal or physiognomic perception. See Graph 1.

---

[3] **All electrical currents are associated with corresponding magnetic fields. On a deeper level, this electromagnetic propogation has a quantum mechanical dimension of partical and wave dynamics, along with other properties. Quantum mechanical dynamics include nonlocality, vibratory interpenetration, possible superconductivity, and a shifting matrix of energy identities and fluxuations arising in the vacuum of "space." This "vibratory dimension" is directly *experienced* or felt in human consciousness in both the purely energetic domain of what we presently call physics and in the spiritual domain of "Presence", such as the Orishas and other forms of evolutionary intelligence. We do not see hear taste or smell gravity, rather we experience its force and its distortion of spacetime. We do not see the Orisha, however the trained devotee feels their vibration and experiences their "force" in their lives.**

It is our suggestion here that neuromelanin provides these "pathways" of internal perception. There are also certain other quantum mechanical entrainment effects of cortical melanin with the wider solar, geogravitational and electromagnetic environment that become focused under specific psycho physiological and cognitive conditions explored in diverse meditative disciplines alluded to earlier (Bynum, in process). When these disciplines are consciously initiated in the attention association areas of the prefrontal cortex they eventually affect the orientation association areas of the brain located in the posterior section of the left and right parietal lobe by what is termed "deafferentation" or the decrease of neural input (Newberg, D'Aquili and Rause, 2002). This gray neuromelanin dense area is located in the top rear section of the brain in what is termed the posterior superior parietal lobe. The sense of space, time, self and psychological boundary limitation is radically affected and thereby the sensation of "travel" or shifting in space, time, and distance is altered. This freeing of the self "reflection" from the conventional structures of space, time and matter then allows this self sense to interact with other neural structures and processes to unfold an atypical but profoundly realized experience.

There is a neuromelanin nerve track strategically embedded in the midbrain limbic system explored later in this text by Richard D King. This Amenta nerve tract is concentrated most significantly in the substantia nigra at the beginning of a kind of loop in the track, and then it "rises up" to the nucleus brachialis pigmentosus, then the nucleus paranigralis to the locus coeruleus, before descending in a long column that extends the length of the brainstem. See chart III. "The column begins in the midbrain, ventral to the somatic motor neurons of the third nerve nucleus, dorsomedial to the substantia nigra, and in contiguity to the nucleus paranigralis. [It ends] at the nucleus retroambigualis. In the remaining sections of the medulla, the column continues moving laterally until it ends in direct continuity with the intermediolateral gray of the cervical spinal cord" (Bazelon and Fenichel, 1967). When we observe this structure we see the gray of this brain constellation then moves down through the brainstem and projects directly down and into the spinal cord itself forming a continuous gray melanin structure interconnected from beginning to end.

Chart III
Recent mapping of the human brain stem has located 12 areas with high concentrations of pigmented cells. (Olszewski, 1964;Olszewski and Baxter, 1954). They are localized around the midline structures near the third and fourth ventricles or cavities. They lay between the brain and its peripheral organs and each communicate in complex ways with the cerebrospinal fluid.

1. Substantia nigra
2. Nucleus brachialis pigmentosus
3. Nucleus paranigralis pedunculopontine
4. locus coeruleus medialis
5. Nucleus intracapularis
6. Nucleus subcoeruleus
7. Nucleus nervi trigemini mesencephalic
8. Nucleus pontis centralis oralis
9. Nucleus tegmental
10. Nucleus parabrachialis
11. Dorsomotor nucleus of the vagus
12. Nucleus retro ambigulais

    Neuromelanin is exceedingly sensitive and receptive to light or luminosity in various modes. Melanin, in its affinity to certain laser characteristics, actually *absorbs* light and these light absorbing melanin pigment vesicles possess both free radical-redox and ion control mechanisms along with the capacity for energy exchange or transformation from state to state by way of photon-phonon transfer processes. It literally reflects an internally perceived bioluminosity. This is true for human beings in diverse cultures and meditative traditions across time. In that context we find here a parallel or complimentarity between an external light or image reflecting some internal "physiognomic" perception of a "current" of inner light that is collectively projected out and expressed mythologically in many ancient cultures and traditions, one example being the symbol of the "all seeing eye of Tibet." This projection outward of an internally perceived process is similar to what we have been calling " physiognomic perception" in developmental psychology (Werner, 1948; Werner and Kaplan, 1963). This awareness seems to have reached a clinical level in the work of the Kemetic Egyptians who were astute medical observers of such phenomena and its relationship to illness. (King.1990) Their term was the "eye" of Horus. The Taoist medical practitioners have developed procedures for the "circulation" of this blissful " eye" or light in major and minor " orbits" through the body along the spinal line. Historically both these disciplines and traditions have coupled these energetic phenomena with other processes in a wider, more nonlocal solar ecology.

These disciplines have operational capacities in the modern world. The eminent anthropologists Marcel Griaule and Germaine Dieterlen (1986) report from the field that the Dogon of Mali, who trace their historical and genetic lineage to pre-dynastic Egypt some 5000 years ago, by using a very similar methodology dating back over 600 years to at least the 13th century, were able to locate, without the aid of telescopes, the dwarf companion star to the star Sirius. The Dogon described its orbital "shape" and duration with precision. They described how it orbits on its own axis and also recognized its unique gravitational characteristics as a very small but dense star. This star, called Sirius B or Digitaria, has a magnitude of 8 and is invisible to the naked eye. It has a revolution around Sirius every 50 years affecting the "shape" of its orbit and possessing elemental contents that mark it as a dense star. It was only first seen by telescope in the " modern scientific world" by two American astronomers, the Alwan Clarks, a father and son team, in 1862 and not actually photographed until 1970 by Irving Lindenblad of the U.S. Naval Observatory. The Dogon also accurately described another flashing object near Sirius B, which has only recently been seen by the NASA Einstein X-ray satellite, which turned out to be a dwarf nova.

The star Sirius is termed sigi tolo by the Dogon, and Digitaria is referred to as po tolo. Digitaria or po tolo is actually a white dwarf or "embryological" star for other stars and is in the constellation of Orion. Sirius and its other satellites are called the ku tolo or " stars of the head", while the others are referred to as gozu tolo or " stars of the body" The Kemetic Egyptians referred to po tolo or Digitaria as the "Sun behind the sun" and represented it as the hawk god Horus enfolding the head of the pharaoh in their statues. Interestingly enough from our perspective here, identification with the position of the po tolo reveals that the world is turning as through on a spiral. There is a spiraling, elliptical shape in the orbits of Sirius and Digitaria, there is a spiraling, serpentine-like shape in the modulating spatial structure between the first and last of the brain neuromelanin foci we are discussing. In other words, there appears to be a configurationally similarity in the "orbits" of the outer world and the inner world. " As above, so below. As within, so without".

Now whether we accept these field reports by Griaule and Dieterlen or not, they express a controversial and contentious debate within science with arguments claiming complete authenticity to others suggesting gross misinterpretation by these Western scientists. These Dogon claims might be dismissed if there was not such a long tradition of other such reports by the ancient scholars and astronomers from Proclus on across a whole spectrum of eras and cultures, the earliest recorded being the Hermes Trismegistic literature where it was referred to as the " Dark Mystery" or the " Black Rite" (Mead, 1964;Temple, 1976). This ancient part of the world records other accurate astronomical observations ranging from the pre-Christian megalithic site at Namoratunga in modern Kenya to the celestial ruins of Nabta Playa eons ago in the distant Nubian Sahara. Such claims often seem to rest on observations of the external world and correlations with the intimate functions of the human body. This suggests a deeper connection. It is quite possible that our current laws of physics on which we implicitly define our concepts and boundaries of mind do not entirely confine the limits of consciousness. Future discoveries may greatly expand our understanding of this "above-below" connection. Our deepest intuition of consciousness will always be intimately associated with our most adventurous conception of light. These long standing and consensually validated observations from the field by noted anthropologists may be due to mere coincidence, to chance. However this now seems more and more remote. There is another possibility, perhaps another epistemology.

Does every tissue of spacetime have enfolded within it in seed form the history and structure of the entire cosmos? As it unfolds would each level or plane of explication in turn manifest a projection, amplification and reverberation of these other progressively more enfolded levels, surfaces and orders? Within the body itself are there planes or surfaces such as the palms of the hands, bottoms of the feet, the ear, tongue or iris of the eyes, where the entire organization of the body can be found and "awakened"? After all there is a bodily representation or sensory homunculus in the sensory cortex of the precentral gyrus and a motor homunculus in the anterior central gyrus on the brain's surface (mostly) as well as a form of motor homunculus configured lower in the mid-brain cerebellum region near the pons. In this interconnected and interpenetrating field of mind, body and brain does each organ system manifest a signature vibratory mode within this system amenable to conscious intervention under certain states of focused observation? And finally, within the intimate convolutions of the brain itself do these vortices and planes of manifestation, like the dynamics of gravity, provide latticework, pathways and extended connectivity to the interwoven loom of space?

It is quite possible that the similarity of these inner and outer orbits in the brain and the physical universe that we *actually feel in states of unitative conscious experience* is due to a similarity awakened through a nonlocal connection such as information exchange or travel through electron tunneling, or by way of a vibratory affinity such as quantum resonance between these brain structures and the "representative space" these stars and other structures move through. In other words there appears to be a hidden algorithmic contiguity between internal and external space created by an interaction between these neuromelanin foci, brain structures in vibration and the topological curvatures of enfolded space[4].

In any event these observations made by the Dogon and celebrated in their ceremonies have stood the test of time and are consensually "validated" by their religious disciplines and recently by modern astronomical science. Regardless of these ancient observations, this orbit or circulation or directly observable current of sensation appears at the very least to reflect this nigrostriatial area of neuromelanin foci in the midbrain limbic system and perhaps reflects the anlage pathway of the brainstem and below that emerged early in embryogenesis through the neural crest guided by the melanin and neuromelanin self-regulating process (Barr, 1983).

It is suggested that when the neuromelanin or nigrostriatial area is only mildly " activated", as in the procedure outlined in this chapter, the internal perception is of a subtle and relaxing luminous circuit or orbit along the

---

[4] Topology is a different type of geometry that lies beyond the classical three-dimensional Euclidean form. Its focus is on intersection, boundary and containment where figures and spaces enclose eachother and holes pass through figural relationships. "Distance" in the classical sense is either not crucial or irrelevant and points of connectivity or convergence can be achieved in an inherently curved space of multiple or "N" dimensions. The three-dimensional world unfolds out of enfolded "N" dimensional geometry. A paradigm most similar is the Kemetic Egyptian Primeval Waters of NUN where the manifest world of forms, forces, objects, and beings unfolds out of the unmanifest vibrational reality of NUN, a quantum sea of light energy beyond the "zero-point energy." Contemporary String theory is also similar in its description of space, time, matter, and gravitation as unfolded from an enfolded ten-dimensional vibrational reality with potentially innumerable other "planes of correspondance" and points of connectivity.

spinal line that parallels the movement or neuromodulation along this column. When this nigrostriatial column however is fully " awakened" by diverse means and disciplines, there is a distinct and intense perception of bioluminosity emerging from this dark matter of the spine up into the brain core and beyond. It is subjectively experienced in the early stages along the spine as an undulating and living force. This may be due to the further resonant and rhythmic entrainment of neuromelanin foci, topologically situated in the third and fourth ventricles of the brain. The other organs in this dark inner chamber are termed the circumventricular organs. This level or "plane" then, by a resonate affinity established by the properties of neuromelanin, would in turn further project, amplify and reverberate up and into the region of the sensory motor cortex in the precentral gyrus accounting for that peculiar circular sensory cortex "current" so often observed in classical meditative experiences (Bentov, 1977: Sannella, 1987).

It is significant to note here for our purposes that these circumventricular organs are midline brain structures that border the third and fourth ventricles and are outside the blood-brain barrier. Because blood and the cerebrospinal fluid flows between structures and fluids more freely here than in other regions of the body and brain, there is a radical increase in communication between these structures, peripheral organs and the blood born products and information at these sites. These circumventricular organs include the pineal gland, median eminence, subfornical organ, area postrema, subcommissural organ, organum vasculosum of the lamina terminalis, and include the intermediate and neural lobes of the pituitary. When these structures are set in motion by orchestrated breathing and concentration and/or ritual dance and coordinated bodily pulsation, or other meditative disciplines, there is a synchronized vibration between the third and the fourth ventricles which are connected by a tunnel of cerebrospinal fluid. When this vibratory spiral reaches the pineal gland, it stimulates it in an upward fashion. The pineal is attached to areas located in the fourth ventricle and floats in this vibrating pool of cerebrospinal fluid. Because neuromelanin has the capacity to transform energy from one state to another, i.e. the photon-phonon transfer process that occurs in a piezoelectric gel where mechanical vibrations are converted into electrical energy, it may supply the energy of this internally perceived "current" that appears to move along on the form of a staff or lower portion of a cross. The stimulated pineal would thereby become the newer and higher plane amplification and reverberation of this initial loop at the top of this

perceived column or staff, and the diagonal or plane of this physiognomic perceived cross presumably would be that area where neuromelanin is most concentrated on the twelve foci tract. This new loop of awakened energy would come to be symbolized as an "eye" or bird or other symbol of light, flight, insight or illumination and freedom.
See chart III and graph 3.

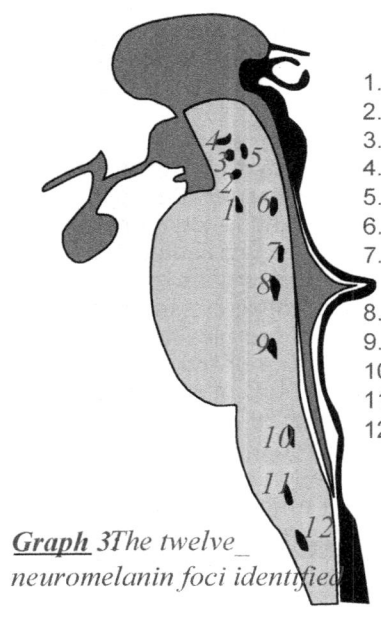

1. Substantia nigra
2. Nucleus brachialis pigmentosus
3. Nucleus paranigralis
4. Locus coeruleus
5. Nucleus intracapularis
6. Nucleus subcoeruleus
7. Nucleus nervi trigemini mesencephalis
8. Nucleus pontis centralis oralis
9. Nucleus tegmental pedunculopontine
10. Nucleus parabrachialis medialis
11. Dorsomotor nucleus of the vagus
12. Nucleus retro ambigualis

Graph 3*The twelve neuromelanin foci identified*

In the later stages when the meditative process had been experienced and fully realized by enough practitioners, the dense "feature detecting" neurons of the limbic system, especially the neocortical surface of the inferior temporal lobe and the amygdala (Joseph, 2000), would physiognomic project outward this luminous closed loop or elliptical cross or ankh that many others would come to recognize as a primordial human process. (Bynum, 1993). This light interacting neuromelanin web and its projections, beginning early in embryogenesis and continuing on through the subsequent stages of development, provides for the latticework of other more subtle bioelectrical pathways through the higher, enfolded cerebral structures of the brain known in the disciplines of meditative reflection but as yet not within the provinces of biomolecular science (Bynum, in process).

Again piezoelectric and other inherent phenomena of biological organisms such as electro-streaming properties, provides for the transduction of energy and information from movement, mechanical stresses, vibration and sound into electromagnetic oscillations. Magnetic fields in particular penetrate through the body and skull with relatively little loss of amplitude and provide for dynamic electrical changes in the process.

For human beings the pineal gland in particular functions not only as a site of photo sensitive processes, but its organ design function and strategic location in a vibrating fluid sea allows it to be an EMF (electromagnetic field) sensor for these magnetic fields and to detect ELF (extremely low frequency) oscillations. These are directly experienced in meditative states and other conditions of focused subjective attention.

The highly ordered water and cellular state of living matter, a nearly crystalline latticework or structure, versus the significantly less well ordered state of non-living systems, makes biological superconductivity (type II) a possibility at room temperature as opposed to the kind of superconductivity (type I) that is observed at extremely low temperatures in non-living systems. Electron pairs flow more freely across small junctures at these quantum mechanical levels of enfolded space such that the usual "space-distance" dimension is less crucial for the communication of information than the " form-resonance" or quantum mechanical tunneling dynamism.

A crucial aspect of this type II or biological superconductivity is that it transmits the magnetic field in multiples or rhythms of unit quantum magnetic flux thereby making the organism potentially sensitive, under certain restricted and disciplined conditions, to extremely subtle magnetic and gravitational fields (Dubrov, 1978). Remember that of the four fundamental forces currently identified in physical nature it is only electromagnetism and gravity that are actually *experienced in human consciousness*. The so called 'strong force' and 'weak force' are confined to the internal structure of the atom .It is known that vast geothermal and magnetic forces within the earth's rotating core dynamics torque upwards and generate an electromagnetic field in discrete lines of force over the surface of the earth. Einstein showed that gravity itself can be understood as an expression of the geometry of space and is woven into the loom of spacetime. Also we remember that electromagnetism and gravity are both experienced through the nexus of human consciousness. It is therefore not unreasonable to include the subtle effect of both internally generated terrestrial magnetism, electromagnetism and external astronomical gravitational fields within this wider topologically complex ecology. A quieted and sensitive nervous system can be made aware of this matrix of subtle but dynamic relationships, both as they emerge from within the earth and as they descend into the earth through and are conducted along subtle lines of force. In states of deep meditation, healing or other forms of contemplative discipline when there is a resonance between the base heart aorta rhythm (roughly 7hz), the earth-ionosphere electromagnetic cavity radiance at multiples of 7.8 hz, termed the Schumann resonance, and wider solar entrainment effects, we enter into unusual states of expanded awareness (Bynum,in process). Under such restricted conditions, psychologically speaking, the loom of spacetime itself appears as mutable as a conscious dream.

These bioelectrical properties of neuromelanin and melanin in the brain and along the brainstem have recently begun receiving a great deal of attention in the clinical literature (McGinness, Corry and Proctor, 1974;McGinness and Proctor, 1973; Barr, 1983). Melanin and neuromelanin, already clearly established as light sensitive semi-conductors, are excellent candidates for the role of neuromodulator of the central nervous system (Longue-Higgins, 1960;Filatous, McGinness and Corry, 1976;Filatous, McGinness and Williams, 1980). Both subtle magnetic fields and their associated bioelectrical currents can be stimulated in the brain which then profoundly affects human consciousness. As this is more and more born out in clinical practice it will revolutionize the life sciences. It brings into possibility the effect of biological superconductivity, a relatively new hypothesis in clinical science. (Little.1965, Cope, 1981; Cope, 1979) One immediately thinks not only of the psycho physiological symptoms already mentioned, but also of symptoms such as seasonal affective disorder (Terman,Terman,Schlager et al, 1990; Light for Better

Living) and other depressive symptoms in addition to symptoms involving decreased subjective energy or under activation of the autonomic nervous system. In terms of understanding the diverse meditative disciplines of the earth's peoples and their connectivity to the wider terrestrial and cosmic ambience, its capacity for unification and a collective psycho spiritual trajectory is beyond our present comprehension.

Conclusion

We have presented a standardized technique for activation of the autonomic nervous system which appears to be intimately associated with the psychophysical and neurodynamics of neuromelanin. This is a procedure that can be taught in a standardized way to patients responding or suffering from acute or prolonged psycho physiological symptomatology. It involves definite and well-known psychophysical and subjective reactions. However beyond these primarily theraputic functions it may also be indicated in clinical and subtle psycho physiological and bioelectrical or superconductive processes which we are only beginning to understand. There even appear to be nonlocal relationships and perhaps topological contiguities between micro neural processes and the macro processes of the cosmos, specifically a configurational similarity between certain brain neuromelanin foci and spiraling constellational structures. We suspect that consciousness may share with quantum mechanics certain general features under restricted conditions, these features being the capacity for trans-temporal and trans-spatial information exchange, or what is termed nonlocality. These are events occurring within the universe of the body and the wider physical universe with which the body interfaces, both of which are interpenetrated by the same principals intimately connecting us all in a more inclusive ecology. What applies to one above or "within" applies to the other below or "without". We look further down the road toward this clinical procedure, which allows us to communicate more directly, and clearly with the body. It offers a great deal of hope to the patient suffering from seemingly intractable pain and illnesses.

REFERENCES

Achterberg, J. and Lawlis, G.F. (1984). Imagery and disease. Champaign, IL: I.P.A.T.

Alternating cerebral hemispheric activity and lateralization of autonomic nervous function. Human Neurobiology, 39-43.

Amaral,D.G. and Sinnamon, H.M., 1977 Locus coeruleus. Neurobiology of a central noradrenergic nucleus. Progress in neurobiology,vol 9,147-196.

Bandler, R. and Grinder, J. (1982). Reframing: neuro-Linguistic programming and the transformation of meaning. Moab, UT: Real People Press.

Barr, E.F. (1983). Melanin: the organizing molecule. Medical Hypotheses, 11 1,1-139.

Barr, F.E. (1983). Melanin: The organizing molecule. Medical Hypotheses, 11:1, 1-39.

Bazelon, M. and Fenichel, G.M. (1967). Studies on neuromelanin. I. A melanin system in the human adult brainstem. Neurology, 17, 512-519.

Bentov,I. (1977). Stalking the wild pendulum: On the mechanics of consciousness.N.Y.: Dutton.

Bogerts,B. 1981, A brainstem atlas of catecholaminergic neurons in man, using melanin as a natural marker. Journal of Comparative Neurology, 197, 63-80.

Bynum, E.B.(1999). The african unconscious:roots of ancient mysticism and modern psychology. NYC:Columbia university,teachers college press.

Bynum, E.B. (1993) Transcending psychoneurotic disturbances. Binghamton, NY: Haworth press.

Bynum,E.B.(in process) Kundalini and the psychobiology of transcendence.

Charney, D.S. and Heninger, G.R. (1986). Abnormal regulation of noradrenergic function in panic disorders. Archives of General Psychiatry, 43, 1042-1054.

Charney, D.S., Heninger, G.R. and Breier, A. (1984). Noradrenergic function in panic anxiety. Archives of General Psychiatry, 41, 751-763.

Cope, F.W. (1979). Remnant magnetization in biological materials and systems as evidence for possible superconductivity at room temperature: A preliminary survey. Physiological Chemistry and Physics, 11, 65-69.

Cope, F.W. (1981). Organic superconductive phenomena at room temperature. Some magnetic properties of dyes and graphite interpreted as manifestations of viscous magnetic flux lattices and small superconductive regions. Physiological Chemistry and Physics, 13, 99-110.

Cotzias, G.C. 1974. Melanogenesis and extra pyramidal diseases, Fed. proc., 23,,713.

Diop, A.C. (1974). The African origin of civilization (M. Cook, Trans.). Westport, CT: Lawrence Hill and Co.

Diop, C.A. (1991). Civilization or barbarism: an authentic anthropology. (Yaa-Lengi Meema Ngemi, Trans.). Brooklyn, NY: Lawrence Hill Books.

Dubrov,A.P. (1978). The geomagnetic field and life : geomagnetobiology (F.L. Sinclair, trans.) New York: Plenum.

Ebbell, B. (1937). The papyrus ebers: the greatest Egyptian medical document (B. Ebbell, Trans.). Copehagen, Levin and Munksgaard.

Edmonston, W.E. (1986). The induction of hypnosis. New York: J. Wiley and Sons.

Elama, M., Svensson, T.H.E., and Thoren, P. (1986). Locus coeruleus neurons and sympathetic nerves: activation by visceral afferents. Brain Research, 375, 117-125.

Erickson, M.H. and Rossi, E.L. (1979). Hypnotherapy: An exploratory casebook. New York: Irvington Publishers, 94-142.

Fenichel, G.M. and Bazelon, M. (1968). Studies on neuromelanin. II. Melanin in the brainstem of infants and children. Neurology, 18, 817-820.

Filatous, G.J., McGuinness, J.E. & Williams, L. (1980). Statistical analysis of switching in melanin. Physiological Chemistry and Physics, 12, 534-538.

Filatous, J., McGinness, J. & Corry, P. (1976). Thermal and electronic contributions to switching in melanins. Biopolymers, 15, 2309-2319.

Finch,C S. 1990 African background to medical science. London: Karnak House.

Foote, S.L., Bloom, F.E. and Aston-Jones, C. (1983). Nucleus Locus coeruleus: new evidence of anatomical and physiological specificity. Physiological Review, 63, 844-914.

Fried, R. (1987). The hyperventilation syndrome: Research and clinical treatment. Baltimore and London: John Hopkins University Press.

Funderbunk, J. (1977). Science studies yoga: a review of physiological data. Honesdale, PA: Himalayan International Institute of Yoga Science and Philosophy.

Gillis, R.A., Quest, J.A. Pagani, F.D. et al (1991). Control centers in the central nervous system for regulating gastroinstestinal motility. In R.A. Gillis, J.A. Quest and F.D. Pagani (Eds.) Handbook of Physiology. New York: Oxford University Press.

Gorman, J.M., Liebowitz, M.R., Fyer, A.J. et al (1989). A neuroanatomical hypothesis for panic disorder. American Journal of Psychiatry, 146, 148-161.

Griaule,M and Dieterlen, G. 1986. The pale fox. Az. Continuum Foundation.

Grinder, L. and Bandler, R. (1981). Trance-formation: Neuro-Linguistic programming and the structure of hypnosis. Moab, UT: Real People Press.

Hassert,D.L.,Miyashita,T. and Williams,C.L. 2004.The effects of peripheral vagal nerve stimulation at a memory modulating intensity on norepinephrine output in the basolateralamygdala. Behavioral Neuroscience.118,vol.1.

Hourning, E. (1986). The discovery of the unconscious in ancient Egypt. Spring: an annual of archetypal psychology and Jungian thought, 16, 28.

Huang Ti (1966). The yellow emperor's classic of internal medicine (I. Veith, Trans.). Berkeley, CA: University of California Press.

Jackson, J.G. (1970). Introduction to African civilization. Secaucus, NJ: Citadel Press.

Joseph R. 2000. The transmitter to god: The limbic system, the soul and spirituality. San Jose, CA: University of California press.

Kagan, J. and Rosenberg, A. (1987). Iris pigmentation and behavioral inhibition. Developmental Psychobiology, 20 (4), 377-392.

Kiecolt-Glaser, J.D., Stephens, R.E. et al (1985). Distress and DNA repair in human lymphocytes. Journal of Behavorial Medicine. 8,311-320.

King, R.D. (1990). The African origin of biological psychiatry. Germantown, TN: Seymore Smith, Inc.

King, R.D. (1990). The question of melanin--the study of blackness [video]. National Association of Black Psychologists, Washington, D.C.

Klein, R. and Armitage, R. (1979). Rhythms in human performance: 1 1/2 hour oscillations in cognitive style. Science, 204, 1326-1328.

Kuvalayananda, S. (1978). Pranayama. Philadelphia, PA: Sky Foundation.

Light for Better Living: The Ultra-Bright Light Systems, Medic-Light, Inc. Yacht Club Drive, Lake Hopatcong, NJ 07849

Little, W.A. (1965). Superconductivity at room temperature. Scientific American, 212 (2), 21-27.

Locke, S. and Colligan, D. (1986). The healer within: The new medicine of mind and body. Bergenfield, NJ: New American Library.

Longue-Higgins, H.C. (1960). On the origin of the free radical property of melanins. Archives of Biochemistry and Biophysics, 86, 231-232.

Lysebeth, A.V. (1983). Pranayama: The yoga of breathing. London, Boson and Sydney: Unwin Paperbacks.

Marsden,C.D.1961. Pigmentation in the nucleum substantiae nigrae of mammals. Journal of anatomy,95,162-256

McGinness, J. and Proctor, P. (1973). The importance of the fact that melanin is black. Journal of Theoretical Biology, 39, 677-678.

McGinness, J., Corry, P. & Proctor, P. (1974). Amorphous semiconductor switching in melanins. Science, 183, 853-855.

Mead, G.R.S, 1964 Thrice greatest Hermes. London: John Watkins Publishers

Meyer, J.S. (1985). Biochemical effects of corticosteroids on neural tissue. Physiological Review, 65 (4), 946-1020.

Moore,T.O. 1995 The science of melanin: dispelling the myths.Silver Spring,MD: Beckham House.

Moore,T.O. 2002 Dark matters,dark secrets. Redan GA:Zamani Press.

Motoyama, H. (1981). Theories of the chakras: Bridge to higher consciousness. Wheaton, IL: Theosophical Publishing House. 142-154.

Muses, C. (1972). Trance-induction techniques in ancient Egypt. In C. Muses and A.M. Young (Eds.) Consciousness and reality: The human pivot point (pp. 9-17). New York: Avon Books.

Netter, F.H. (1972). The CIBA collection of medical illustrations, Vol. 1, The nervous system. Summit, NJ: CIBA Press.

Newberg,A.,D'Aquili,E. and Rause,V 2002 Why god won't go away. New York,NY: Ballantine Books

Olszewski,J. 1964. Cytoarchitecture of the human brain. N.Y., Stern and Birjelow.

Olszewski,J. and Baxter,D. 1954 Cytoarchitecture of the human brain stem. Basel and N.Y.,S. Karger.

Prakashan, P. (1980). Shiva Svarodaya, Varanasi, India: Chowkhamba Sanskrit Series.

Rama, S. (1981). Application of sushumna (Cassette Recording No. 0308). Honesdale, PA: Himalyan International Institute of Yoga Science and Philosophy.

Rama, S., Ballentine, R. and Hymes, A. (1979). Science of breath. Honesdale, PA: Himalayan International Institute of Yoga Science and Philosophy.

Rider, M.S., Achterberg, J., Lawlis, G.F., et al (1990). Effect of immune system imagery on secretory IgA. Biofeedback and Self-Regulation, 15 (4), 317-333.

Sannella,L.(1987). The Kundalini experience : psychosis of transcendence. Lower Lake,CA;Integral Publishing.

Scherer,H.J.1939. Melanin pigmentation of the substantia nigra in primates. Journal of comparative anatomy,71,91-95.

Siever, I.J., Uhde, T.W., Jimerson, D.C. et al (1984). Differential inhibitory noradrenergic responses to clonidine in 25 depressed patients and 25 normal control subjects. American Journal of Psychiatry, 141, 733-741.

Sperry, R.W. (1988, August). Psychology's mentalist paradigm and the religion/science tension. American Psychologist, 607-612.

Svatmarama, S. (1971). The shambhavi mudra and the inner light. In The yoga of light: Hatha yoga pradipika, (H. Rieker and E. Becherer, Trans.). Middletown, CA: Dawn House Press. 164-175.

Temple,R.K.G.,1976. The Sirius Mystery Camberwell,London: Sidgwick & Jackson,Ltd.

Terman, J.S., Terman, M., Schlager, D., et al (1990). Efficacy of brief, intense light exposure for treatment of winter depression. Psychopharacology Bulletin, 26 (1), 3-10.

Thakkur, C.G. (1977). Yoga: Harmony of body, mind and soul. 375 Kalbadeui Road, Bombay, India: Yoga research Center/Ancient Wisdom Publications.

Tokay, E. (1972). Fundamentals of physiology. New York: Barnes and Noble.
Warner,H. and Kaplan ,B. 1963. Symbol formation .NY: J. Wiley and sons.

Werner,H. 1948 Comparative psychology of mental development. NY: international universities press.

Werntz, D. (1981). Cerebral hemisphere activity and autonomic nervous function. Unpublished doctoral dissertation, University of California, San Diego.

Werntz, D., Bickford, R., Bloom, F. and Shannahoff-Khalsa, D. (1981, February). Selective cortical activation by alternating autonomic function. Paper presented at the Western EEG Society Meeting, Reno, Nevada.

CHAPTER 4

NEUROMELANIN: A BLACK GATE THRESHOLD; THE I33 TISSUE OF HERU, HISTORICAL, NEUROPSHYSIOLOGICAL AND CLINICAL PSYCHOLOGICAL ISSUES

BY

RICHARD D. KING, M.D.

Introduction

"O Wosir the King, take the Eye of the living Heru that you may see with it. O Wosir the King, may your vision be cleared by means of the light. O Wosir the King, may your vision be brightened by the dawn.O Wosir, the King, I give to you the Eye of Heru when Ra gives it. O Wosir the King, I put forth to you the Eye of Heru on that you may see with it".
Utterance 639,(Faulkner,1969)Pyramid Texts,3200-2100 B.C.E Kemetic Old Kingdom

Scope, Methods and Issues

This chapter will review the subject of neuromelanin for several issues that are related to (1) the history of the ancient African study of Black symbolism/melanin/neuromelanin; (2) the current era's scientific study of concepts related to neuromelanin; (3) the role of neurogenesis or new nerves as they are added to the cortex and affected by psychosocial stressors and (4) current era concepts of the clinical practice of psychology/psychiatry related to neuromelanin anatomy and physiology. The methodology is one of clinical psychiatry ,which focuses on the use of dynamic symbolism, ontological meaning and emotional-historical context in the analysis and understanding of human motivation, behavior and consciousness. Dynamic symbolism is a reflection of internal processes and has the capacity to transform and heal the body and mind when intelligently focused and understood. It is therefore critical in this light that a study of neuromelanin be seen as a study that is an integral part of a much larger study of melanin, not only skin melanin, but brain melanin in the classical and historical tradition of melanin as the Kemetic flesh of Ra, (Piankfoff, 1954). The neurocosmological implications of the Black carbon atom and especially Black cosmic melanin/nanodiamonds of carbon-rich proto-planetary nebulae interstellar Black matter, is also implicated in this wider view that embraces both the micro-worlds within us and the cosmic ambience that dwells about us. For as surely as this is one universe, the inner and outer aspects of it must interpenetrate and meet at some level of manifestation. This is indeed the whole thrust of the ancient vision on the banks of the Nile in Kemet and the root of our modern concept of it as neurocosmology.(Van Kerekhoven, 2002; Hill, 1998; Luu, 1993; Bradley, 1966; Liou 1996; Nicolaus, 1998; B. Nicolaus, 1997; R. Nicolaus, 1997).

Melanin, Nanodiamonds and the Lineage of Panspermia

The cosmic carbon atom interstellar gas clouds of nanodiamonds/cosmic melanin and their relationships to biological melanin and neuromelanin is a fundamental category of knowledge that yields a critical meaning to a study of melanin which dismisses the two tendencies in modern science that seek for ideological reasons to lessen the impact of melanin studies. One tendency is to dismiss melanin studies simply as pseudoscience. This is to equate and associate melanin with the mere waste products of cellular metabolism. Is melanin a biological waste product or a luminous jewel waiting to be rediscovered and understood by us in modern times.(B. Nicolaus, 1998)? Clearly, the absurdity of such a devaluation of melanin studies is made readily apparent by the intuitive knowledge that interstellar Black matter in the form of interstellar gas clouds laden with these luminous jewels of Black nanodiamonds are the literal genetic seeds from which stars are born. They arise from the same high-energy primordial shock and flux that populated all of creation. In this paper we are openly suggesting that there truly is a crucial connection between the black or dark matter that structures much of the unseen universe and the subtle living dark matter that structures our very bodies, brains and nervous systems. The study of higher order mathematics, physics and chemistry that observe such cosmic melanin macrocosmic phenomena should be a wake up call that a similar higher science is required to study carbon/melanin related to microcosmic phenomena in living biosystems on planet Earth, i.e. humanity. Is inner melanin in some as yet unknown way a gateway to the outer world dark matter? Where does this black material so intimately associated with life itself come from in the first place?

The interstellar material of our Milky Way galaxy contains in a huge state vast interstellar gas clouds composed of hydrogen (70%) and helium (28%) with a small component of a solid particles, interstellar or cosmic dust.(Nicolas,2002). In addition to the element carbon there has been found in the interstellar expanses the elements oxygen, nitrogen, nickel, sulfur, aluminum, iron and others along with many different organic and inorganic molecules. It is believed that following the initial so called Big Bang of creation that the universe expanded in a hot burst of pure energy then later cooled down into the condensation of the early subatomic quark soup leading to the first elements hydrogen .Stars were formed by this process which initially were mostly hydrogen The processes of gravitational collapse and other cosmic forces eventually created a nuclear fusion state that fused the nucluei of hydrogen atoms together to produce helium atoms. The helium then continued to fuse producing atoms of progressively higher atomic number, nucluei with more protons and neutrons fusion where internal heat gradually increased and transformed the structure of gas particles. It is out of this flux of "mother" gas clouds that the carbon atom arose. This is a vast simplification of a complex process but the point is a critical end product of black nanodiamonds of carbon.. Van Kerekhoven(2002) reported that the temperature, pressure and composition/molecular precursors in the solar nebula would favor the condensation of carbonaceous compounds, what are called nanodiamonds. Diamond formation is favored by an abundance of atomic hydrogen and low carbon ratios. Nanodiamonds are a common by product of star formation regions formed in stellar sytems and ejecta from a supernova carbon star explosion.

Meteorites containing interstellar diamonds were first reported in 1989(Lewis,1989). The extra-solar origin of the nanodiamonds was indicated by isotopic anomalies of 15n depletions,P and R Xe compositions, and enhancements of D/H ratios (Anders,1993).Different models of the origin of meteoritic nanodiamonds have been reviewed (Van K,2002; Anders,1993) ranging from interstellar shocks (Tielens,1987) ,to formations in exotic stellar locations (Jorgenson, 1988), to the quantum heating of carbonaceous grains (Nuth,1992).

Nanodiamonds are a solid crystalline form of mostly carbon atoms that are extremely small in size, with median size of~ 3nm (Lewis, 1989; Daulton,1996). This is a size that is ten to one thousand times smaller than interstellar grains (Van Kerckhoven,2002). Nanodiamonds have a large surface area to volume ratio with an active surface chemistry (Hill,1998). It is the nanodiamond's active surface chemistry that results in the formation of active species such CH, CH2, CO, and NH (Hill, 1998). A critical role is served by nanodiamonds and interstellar gas clouds in the formation of stars but also in the creation of biogenetic molecules of melanin in these interstellar clouds in many galaxies and continues to do the same in our solar system, perhaps at the same time that the solar system was created. It is through these interstellar gas clouds that these black biogenetic surfaces, sometimes transported on the larger surfaces of traveling comets along with amino acids, moved through the stellar abyss and throughout the innumberable solar systems seeding the surface of planets like our planet earth.. This is the ancient "panspermia" hypothesis and vision reinterpreted by Nobel laureate Francis Crick and Leslie Orgel (Jantsch, 1980). It is these Black matter melanin seeds from the stellar expanses that provide the biogenetic spark of life. From this perspective it is difficult to see how this material could ever be conceived as mere "waste matter".

Science, Memory And The Amenta

There is a second tendency that continues to lessen the scientific impact of melanin studies and that is one that equates high levels of human melanin skin content with racial inferiority (Jablonski, 2000: Kershaw, 1998; Kershaw, 1999; Guderian, 1952) .Yet every clinician and social scientist of this century knows that for historical reasons over the last 500 years there is a painful relationship between the devaluation of people with high levels of melanin in their mere surface skin pigmentation and the psychology of white supremacy/racism (Welsing, 1970; Welsing, 1990; Ani, 1994). Again, a firm grasp of advanced knowledge in the fields of psychology, neuroanatomy, neuroanatomical embryology, neuropharmacology and historical epigenetic unfoldment are absolutely required to appreciate the deeper dynamic role of melanin in human experience. There are the PTSD or post-traumatic stress disorder psychological emotional trigger effects of visual images of Black symbolism that evoke the outpouring of emotion laden memory projections from within the human mind-. These are the levels or the multiple gates of the Kemetic Amenta, the superconscious, personal unconscious, lower unconscious, and the collective unconscious, all of which are manifestations and projections of the ancient Kemetic understanding of the Primeveal waters of Nun (Assagioli, 1965; Bynum, 1984; Bynum, 1999; King, 1994).

Today's human mind is pregnant with millions, if not billions, of years of emotional, intense active memories of the whole spectrum of ones blood line genetic ancestors. These experiences form a literal ocean of incredible beauty of human experience that range from heaven to hell, from the heights of love, romance and creative genius through the lows of fear, jealousy and post traumatic stress disorder (PTSD). This great phylogenetic storehouse of collective memory even includes our fragmented memories of exposure to geological catastrophes. This is an ocean of living memories of the tragic conversion of the lush watery filled grasslands of North Africa into today's largely barren Sahara desert, Eurasian Glacial ice ages, floods, meteor strikes, earthquakes, and volcanic eruptions; and the countless wars of ethnic cleansing. Amid these however are also those quiet islands of the triumphs of human cooperation, communication and compassion in the interests of mutual survival and evolution toward some higher purpose and union. This has been an epic saga and struggle of hominid evolutionary consciousness from the early australopithecines of pre-antiquity up to the Homo Sapiens Sapiens of today (Bynum, 1999).

Deeper yet, there is in this continuum of living history the current era's oppressive paradigm of white supremacy/racism, that is born from a very great fear of melanin Blackness and of a melanin death/sleep that ironically arises from the comical reality of a missed opportunity, a closed door, a tragic, aborted unfolding or non opening of the psychospiritual door to the higher order melanin structured biophysical systems of luminious blackness. The psychotic yet comical reality of white supremacy witnesses a failure of" growing up", a failure to evolve from a neophyte strictly logical left brain stage of consciousness, to the second stage, a stage of intelligence with inner vision and a dual cortical hemispheric integration, then further on to the third stage of sons/daughters of light, unity of light itself with a Christ consciousness level of inner vision, the perfected human incarnation of biophysical evolution. Thus, white supremacists and their victims of white supremacy experience a horrific tragedy of lowered standards for human potential, a failed adult human transformation in the alchemical bath of life in which the head of the Ethopian is the vessel black philosopher's stone, the Anu Benben stone, melanin/neuromelanin I33 brainstem spinal column which is the threshold door through which such transformations are born.

There are melanin systems that transform the seemingly inert Black earth into the Black diamond of inner vision (King, 1993; Budge, 1967; Faulkner, 1967; Faulkner, 1978; Piankoff, 1977). Inner vision is an advanced science, a disciplined form of introspection, not a form of regression to pre-scientific thinking or pseudoscience. Humanity as yet is only in the anteroom of the next stage of our evolutionary drama. The obscuring Blackness holds the key to the hidden light of inner vision.

Historical Issues in the Ancient African study of Black Symbolism/Melanin/Neuromelanin

African scientists seeking a Black consciousness throughout the past several million years, if not countless ages, have deeply studied nature's script of Black symbolism (James, 1954; Diop, 1991; Clarke, 1999; Allen,

1974; Jackson, 1970; King, 1994; Faulkner, 1969; Faulkner, 1978; Churchward, 1913; Churchward, 1921). Skin melanin, which ancient Egyptians referred to as the "Flesh of Ra" (Piankoff, 1954) and, "I33 Tissue of Horus"(Piankoff, 1977), neuromelanin has been a part of such a study. Neuromelanin is a Black biopigment that is present in neuro or brain tissue including the outer coverings of the brain, dura mater and pia mater (Hyshaw, 1994) and the substance of the brain neurons and glial cells.

This brief history of ancient African study melanin/neuromelanin will concern 5 issues- (1) the Kemetic root name, M3NW, for melanin, (2) pre dynastic Kemetic Memphite cosmology concept of the Hill (Ptah/mind), (3) Kemetic architectural symbolism of the Black Rose Granite Threshold stone, (4) Kemetic architectural symbolism of the Black Rose Granite all Black Kings chamber in the Great Pyramid at Ghiza, and (5) Kemetic statements of neuroanatomy from 1349 B.C. on the right panel second shrine in the Tomb of Tutankamnen.

The history of the ancient African study of melanin begins with the name itself, melanin. The history of the name melanin is that it is an English word derived from the Greek word melan, which means Black (Bernal, 1991). Bernal reported, "there is no common Indo-European root for the color black...however, it would seem more plausible to derive this from the Egyptian (Kemetic) name. M3NW, the mountain in the West; where the sun goes down in the evening, and entrance to the underworld." The Egyptians, here after referred to as Kamites, inherited from Khui land and later Ethiopian ancestors (King,1990; 1994) the M3NW concept. The M3NW concept was part of a philosophical system that witnessed a daily, 24-hour cycle of daylight and night time, in which the sun was seen at sunset to enter the earth at a M3NW (melanin). Manu, gate at a Western Mountain of the Moon,Baku, undergo a 12 hour night time passage through the all Black domain of Amenta with 12 gates and then to emerge at the dawn of morning through an eastern M3NW (melanin) gate, at the Eastern Mountain of the Moon for the 12 hour passage of the sun during daylight.

The extreme antiquity of millions of years of the M3NW root name for melanin is readily apparent. Consider the fact that the geographical place in Africa where the 24-hour day is equally divided into 12 hours of day and 12 hours of night is at the equator of the planet. Moreover, it is at the equatorial region that there are not only ancient African records of an Eastern Mountain of the Moon, Bakhu Kenya's Mount Kiliminjaro (Ben

Jochannan, 1972) but also a Western Mountain of the Moon, Uganda's Mount Renzori, Mountain Range,Manu (Halet). In fact Ben Jochannan (1972) cited the records of the papyrus of Hunefer that stated that, "we Kamites came from the Mountain of the Moon (Kiliminjaro Ethiopians)." Moreover, there are abundant records of Egyptian references to the Great Lake region between the Eastern Mountain of the Moon and Western Mountain as the sites of origin of River Hapi. This source of the Nile is the abode of oldest Egyptian God, Bes, an Anu-Twa person from the Great Lakes region of Khui Land with one group of Anu gathered around the Bakhu eastern mountains of the Moon and another group of Anu ancestors gathered around the Manu western mountain of the moon.

Certainly, it will require advanced studies in multiple fields of study of science, physics, electromagnetism, neurochemistry and music to answer the great scientific questions that our misperception and ignorance now mislabels as pseudoscience. We must explore the questions of what special and perhaps unknown energetic fields relationship exists at the equator of this planet that promote epigenetic unfoldment of upright, walking biological systems called consciously evolving humans.

Budge has written (Budge, 1969) "Bes (The God Bes) has the same type of face as the Pygmy...the earliest mythology of old Egypt, and no doubt Bes, was at the later date made to represent a type of Horus I (Jesus), who was at first their "Chief of the Nome". It was from these Anu (Pygmies) that the first mythology of Egypt sprung". The mythology was humanities first use of verbal, the spoken word, symbolic body-postures (signs, the seen word), rhythmical song/dance (the emotionally/harmonically expressed word), and later written records of deep, emotionally charged memories of the past experiences of blood-line genetic ancestors. Thus current records have confirmed the common origin of all humanity from the same Khui Land Great Lakes origin in North East Africa from before 7 million years ago and subsequent later migrations East into Ethiopia, North to Egypt into Eurasia, South-to-South Africa or West to Chad and West Africa and North Africa. Current anthropological records confirm that the first 5 or more of the past 7 million years was in Africa with only the last 2 years of hominid ancestors migrations outside of Africa beginning with homo erectus. The current branching of the hominid line, our Homo Sapien Sapien family is only roughly 200,000 years. This stock again originated in Africa and then migrated out of Africa onto every continent of the planet. The Amenta that is remembered here is composed of that ocean of common multimillion-year experiences of our ancient common bloodline ancestors, the root bloodline of all humans regardless of surface skin pigmentation. We are all Africans in our bones and genes.(Bynum,1999,Bruwet, 2002; Wood, 2000; Leakey, 1995; Kimbel, 1994; Kappelman, 1996; Asfaw, 1999; Tobias, 1987; Leigh, 1992; Falk, 2000; McHenry, 1998; Reed, 1997; Skelton, 1992).In fact the Anu were the first humans to travel "into" the earth, the first humans to become conscious of the domains and doors within their own unconscious, the first to map Amenta, and in their mythology of the Travel of the Great Hero, Ife, developed a stellar mythos over 2,000,000 B.C.E. (Halet);King,1992;Chruchward,1913;Chruchward,1924).

Involution and Evolution: The Dark Matter Cycles of Spirit and Cosmogenesis

According to James (James, 1954) there exists predynastic records from before the times of Dynastic Kemet (4,000 B.C.). This was the Memphite Theology of the Primate of the Gods. Ptah,who first arose as a prominent hill from the water of Nun, an island in the primeval lake in Khuiland (Chruchward, 1913) or multidimensional vibrational space. The primeval hill arising from the waters of Nun are symbolic metaphors for the mythological summary of our ancestor's conscious intellectual experiences as they progressed from the collective unconscious womb of African root hominid consciousness itself. This is an epigenetic upward pull of the super conscious, the ascension of individual/group life force following an earlier descent of light through space into matter, gravitational condensation of Black nanodiamond interstellar laden gas clouds into proto-stars. It is the involution of spirit down into matter and the evolution of matter back into spirit in the great cycle of Divine manifestation as seen in the sublime vision of Abydos.

From a cosmogenetic perspective we witness the main sequence of star evolution as a star with a carbon core initial stage, flowering to a supernovae seeding of interstellar gas clouds with carbon, through a self organization of complex carbon based organic molecules in interstellar space particularly hydrated water laden comet bodies coated with surface organic molecular-to the seeding of planetary surfaces with living organic dark matter. This self organizing ,biophysical carbon rich molecular unfoldment moves progressively through evolution up through the Mineral Kingdom, Plant Kingdom, and Animal Kingdom to the human species and beyond. Thus, the Kemetic hill can be seen, as a symbol of an erect individual human being as a progressive epigenetic unfoldment.

"As above, so below": Inner Brain Structures and Outer Symbolic Forms

In Kemet the oldest site of the study of the Sun-god was the city of ANU,

> Anu, 🏛️⊙, *i.e.*, The cult of the standing stone, or pillar, was probably older than the cult of Rā, and the old name of Heliopolis is Anu, 🏛️⊙, *i.e.*,

later named Heliopolis by the Greeks and Romans, and named ON in the Christian bible. According to Budge(Budge,1923) it was at ANU that from time immemorial there existed a temple dedicated to the Sun-god and this same temple was supported by an ancient college of priest/scientists who from a very remote period were renown for their wisdom and learning. Critically, ANU is also the name of the ancient Twa people of Africa, related to the early Homo erectus, who over 2 million years ago migrated from the Khui land great lake regions to Ethiopia, Egypt and into every continent. Thus the seminal ideas and concepts of the African Kemetic priests of ANU is a reflection of the germination of these ideas over several million years of the study of the sun, light and the various forms of light to matter. These priests called their god or sun god Tem or Atem and the supremacy of Tem was defined in the various versions of the Book of the Coming Forth by Day(Book of the Dead) in the 17th chapter " I am Tem in his rising. I was the only one.I came into existence in Nenu(Nu, Nun, space). I am Ra when he rose for the first time. I am the great god who created himself from Nenu, and who made his names to become the gods of his company. I am Tem, the dweller in his disk or Ra in his rising in the eastern horizen of the sky. I am yesterday; I know today. I am the Bennu(Black Phoenix) which is in ANU , and I keep the register of the things which are not yet in existence.." These ancient scientists at the old Kemetic university of ANU defined Tem as a man god who absorbed the qualities of earlier African conceptions such as Heru-ur, the old sky god, sun by day between sunset and sunrise, Heru-Khuti,(Horus in the two horizons); Khepra, the sun during the hour that precedes the dawn; and Tem, the setting sun. Thus in the 17th chapter of the book of the Coming Forth by Day, the earlier image of the sun god Tem showed the image of the sun god Ra. Budge noted the importance of the priest scientists of ANU concept of Ra was clearly shown in the III-IV dynasty by the use of the name of Ra of the Neso bat names of the builder of the second   Khaf-Ra)/Khephren and third pyramid (Menkaru-Ra/Myercinus) at Gizah. It was from this same father Tem god later named Ra, earlier named Ptah that presided over the company of others phases of god, light, in the forms of Shu, Tefnuti, Geb, Nut, Osiris (Wosir) , Isis, Set and Nepthys.

    The Kemetic pyramid text from the Kemetic old kingdom from before 5000 years ago does record the ancient ANU African scientist concept related to melanin, neuromelanin in the concept of the black stone, Ben-stone, of rose granite. In the pyramid text, II,N.663,p.372, there is written how the spirit of the sun visited the temple of the sun from time to time in the form of a Black Bennu bird, and alighted" on the Ben-stone, in the house of the Bennu in ANU".

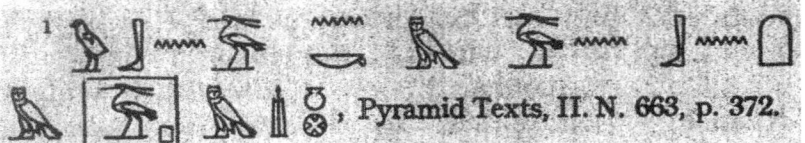

The Bennu bird was known by the Kemetic priests at ANU as the soul of Ra or the Bennu Bird (Phoenix bird). This was a symbolic model of the human Anu form in which light entered the bird like 3rd ventricle, House of the Bennu, threshold cerebrospinal fluid brain system and lighted, and thereby became activated there in the Ben-stone of neuromelanin, in the Black dot, locus coeruleus by the light activation and Black neuromelanin threshold translation of light along the entire 12 gate/12 black nucleui of the black neuromelanin amenta tract, the Kemetic I33 tissue of Horus of the human brain C.S.F. ventricular system, brainstem and spinal column.

Last, we so clearly see the common African origin of all humanity in our common Anu root ancestral viewing of the primordial images of Osiris, Khenti, Amenti and triune god of Osiris of the Osirian resurrection including Seker, the old Death god of Memphis (Budge, 1923).

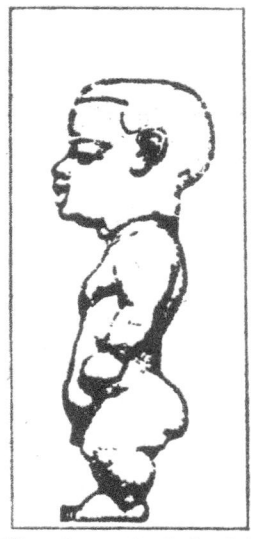

The triune god of the Osirian Resurrection. The three members of his triad were Seker, an old Death-god of Memphis; Ptaḥ, a Creation-god of Memphis; and Osiris, the vivifier of the dead.

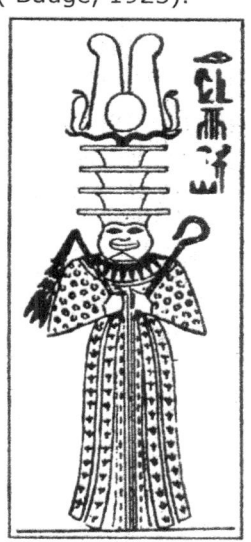

Osiris Khenti Amentt, god and judge of the dead and lord of the Other World.

Accordingly, one must also consider the meaning of the architectural symbolism of the Great Pyramid of Ghiza in Egypt. This is a structure that contains an upper most all black room of Black Rose Granite, the so called Kings chamber that sits directly above the Queens chamber. For if the Great Pyramid is a symbolic model of the erect human form. It is a comparable to the watery all black room , third ventricle,located in the midbrain limbic system structures of human brain.

Another clue to the symbolic meaning of the all Black Rose Granite Room of the King's chamber can be found in the architectural symbolism of the all Black Rose Granite in the temple of Abydos. In this case, Black Rose Granite was used as the bottom, or the threshold stone of the four-sided gate/door entrance into the temple from the outside world into the outer courtyard. This same Black Rose Granite was also seen as the bottom or threshold stone in the four-sided gate/door between the outer courtyard and inner courtyard.

This Black Rose Granite was clearly seen over 5,000 years before the current era functioning as a threshold, or symbolically transformative gateway threshold. Moreover, it was known that there was something black in the heads of humans that was not just a threshold for one line of movement, but was black on all sides and a gateway to 360° expansion of human consciousness, a Black hypercube of unseen planes coming into vibratory manifestation if you will. This has historic and dynamic allusions to awakening, to flight, to the mysteries of transformation and translation. The Islamic holy stone or Kabaa at Mecca is a black cube believed to have fallen from the stellar abyss and capable of completely transforming the human spirit that will burn its dross in the fires of meditation and purification.

Furthermore, upon close, visual inspection of Black Rose Granite, one can clearly observe a Black Stone with numerous streaks, zig zag lines of red, as if it were electricity; energy or light being born out of blackness. This is the luminous Blackness alluded to before. This is the symbolic meaning of the Kemetic scientists who intentionally used such a stone clearly as a threshold entrance to the temple of Abydos, the site where the head of the perfect Black God of Amenta, Wosir was buried in this Kemetic Holy land. Was this the symbolic meaning behind the use of the same Black Rose Granite in the Kings chamber of the Great Pyramid?

Last, of great relevance come the inscriptions of the upper register of the right panel from the 2nd shrine from the tomb of Pharaoh Tutankhamen (Piankoff, 1977; Wimby-Jones,1982).

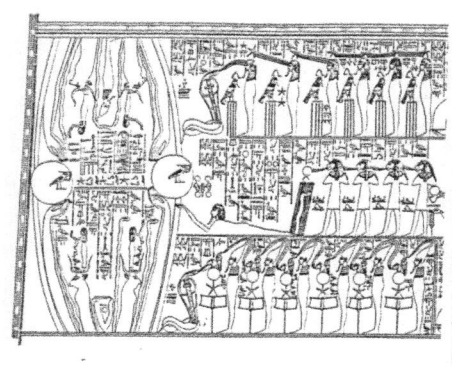 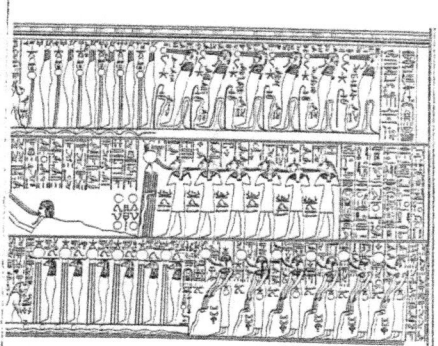

Upper Register-First group of Divinities
(1) The morning (2) The Praiser (3) The Opener (4) The Keres (5) The Incomplete Onc (6) The Corruptible Flesh

Second Group of Divinities
(2) Head of Horus (2) Face of Horus (3) Neck of Horus (4) I 33 Tissues of Horus (5) Inner Eye (6) The Doorway

Third Group of Divinities
(3) Submerged one (2)? (3) Ejaculator (4) Inundator (5) Babe in swaddling cloth (6) The morning bark of Ra

These are critical references to the luminious dark living melanin system present in the head that has come down intact to the present era from the pre-"white" supremacy time of the 18th dynasty, 1349 B.C.

First, the upper registry first group of divinities clearly pictures a star passing rays of light into the midforehead site location of the pineal gland, the site of the light sensitive inner eye, where the hormone serotonin during daylight, and during night, with star light/moonlight, the hormone melatonin is released .Its release has the effect of increasing the activity of melanin systems throughout the body.

Second group of divinities, 3rd figure, named the Neck of Horus, may define the site of the human vocal cords, the site of the production of the spoken word and especially the song word. This site of song production, of human music, defined the ancient study of the role of music and of harmonic resonance in elevating melanin systems, and evoking the soul ascension through harmonic sound (Janata, 2002; Zatorre, 2002).

Third second group of divinities, 4th figure, I 33 tissues of Horus is a clear reference to the spinal cord with 33 vertebrae, which when stood erect I, has a top most part, the head lateral eyes, atop an erect spinal column and the bottom that stands atop a level with the gonads, rectum, and genital organs, the womb of life.

Fourth second group of divinities, fifth figure inner eye, is a clear reference to the pineal gland, an actual phylogentetic 3rd and 4th eye in lower vertebrae, and the eye of inner vision in humans, the posterior floor of the third ventricle.

Fifth second group of divinities, 6th figure, The Doorway, is again a reference to the mystery that there in the head there is a doorway. Sixth, and last, the third group of divinities, the 6th figure, morning bark of Ra, may be a deeper aspect of the doorway in that as the doorway ascends it becomes a vessel of vast travel, a literal star ship, the morning bark of Ra, a black star gate of inner vision. Thus following a review of the right panel, second register from Pharaoh Tutankhamens tomb there is evidence to suggest that the Black room; the King's chamber of the Great Pyramid, was symbolic of a black chamber in the brain of humans that is a doorway ,that is to say a threshold entered into by the eye of inner vision that allows vast ascension; star travel; the morning Bark of Ra, the perfect one, the goal of unity with the light. (Blackshaw,1999; Kume,1999; Pickard,1982; Moore,1995).

Again throughout the shrines of Tut Ankh-Amon there are many reference to Tut Ankh-Amon as the ruler of Helioplois of the south. This clearly defines that the authors of the texts of the shrines were the great and very old college of priests/scientists of Heliopolis, Anu of ancient Anu ancestry, an ancient tradition of African scholarship in the study of psychology.

CURRENT AREAS OF SCIENTIFIC STUDY OF MELANIN AND NEUROMELANIN

The current era has found several eras of scientific study that have added much to our understanding of the meaning and function of both melanin and neuromelanin. These are the areas of physics, anatomy, embryology, endocrinology and psychopharmacology. From physics McGinness (McGinness, 1974) reports on both natural melanin, isolated from melanosomes from a human melanoma at autopsy and synthetic melanin's produced by enzymatic action of mushrooms tyrosine's In both cases when exposed to an electrical current melanin demonstrated the properties of the threshold switching of an amorphous semiconductor. The electrical properties of all the melanin preparations were essentially the same. Threshold switching refers to the ability of Black melanin to switch from an "off" state of low conduction to an "on" state of high conduction of electrical conduction (semi conductor). Furthermore, McGinness, in 2001 Post Publications noted (2001), "...another missed opportunity-melanin's give a flash of light when they switch-clearly electroluminescence, though we did not completely understand its significance at the time".

Again, one can more than marvel at the ancient African use of the Black Rose Granite in the threshold bottom of the Gate/Door entrance to the temple of Abydos. Could the Black Rose Granite which contains flecks of red have been placed in the threshold to symbolize the essential function of melanin as a threshold that under certain energetic conditions switches to high levels of energy, information conduction, and while doing so, simultaneously radiates light into other dimensions (electroluminescence)?

Water hydration was reported to play a critical role in the ability of melanin samples to undergo threshold switching. If the samples were dried for 30 minutes at 200°C they would not switch until rehydrated and dried at room temperature. Water was found to lower the activation energy to conduction by altering the local electric constant of the material. The conductivity of the dopa melanin and isolated melanosomes was found to be high 10.5 (ohm cm) with a resistance of 104ohms for a sample 1 mm thick. The conductivity in the "on" state was increased by a factor of 100 to 1,000. Melanins were found to switch at 3.5 x IG2 volt/cm and through at least 1 cm of material. As a result of these findings McGinness reported that the threshold semi conductor role of melanin was evident in the appearance of melanin in living organisms at locations where energy conversion or charge transfer occurs (the skin, retina of the eye, mid brain structures of the limbic system and the inner ear).

From a neurophysiological perspective, one can appreciate the physiological function of
Neuromelanin. Wherever it is found in its multiple anatomical sites it serves in the role of energy threshold, that is to say of actual "energy conversion" or threshold change transfer.

In the lateral eyes the same threshold role of melanins is seen at the site of retinal-pigmented epithelium. (RPE). One form of charge transfer is the conversion of rod or cone vision pigments entrapped external world photons into an electrical charge for passage into the optic nerve. Another threshold role is the transfer of the rod/come visual pigment carrier of the photons of light signal into a RPE peptide signal, melanoprotein, and a neuroendocrine signal. The melanoprotein signal then is carried through the blood to a mid brain site, the suprachiasmatic nucleus, SCN, in the wall of the 3rd ventrticle. This melanoprotein signal triggers the SCN to pour forth through the L.C. the 12 neuromelaninated nucleui of the Amenta nerve tract I33 Tissue of Horus, pours forth a vast waterfall like cascade of hormonal effects in the 24-hour cycle of the circadian rhythm. This is a 24-hour cycle has a 12-hour rise to a high level of these hormone followed by a 12 hour of decline to a low level of these hormones produced by most of the endocrine glands, and other organ systems of the entire body. It is this environmental light photon/ RPE melanoprotein/ SCN/LC-Amenta trance circadian rhythm that is believed to be so clearly illustrated of the fact that melanin is a threshold door that allows the microcosmic individual human being to be in rhythm with the external macrocosmic world light/dark cycles of environmental lighting.

Neuromelanin in Embryogenesis: The Unfoldment of the Organ Systems

When we return to the enigma of the all black chamber in the inner brain structures, we should remember our neuroembryology and the neuroanatomy as we developed in the womb. First, the biological history of the neuromelanin all black chambers of the brain begin before conception. Melanin is present in the tail of the father's spermatozoa. Melanin is present in the eggs of the mother in her ovary. The egg following release from the ovary is fertilized, united with the spermatozoa in the mother's fallopian tube. The fertilized ovum becomes a rapidly multiplying ball of cells that within hours develops into a ball of cells, the morula, named a morula or blackberry because it looks like a black berry. The outer layer, the cells of the ectoderm, is black. The future epidermal cells maintain their critical relationship to melanin as a site of threshold of energy conversion and/or threshold of change transfer .The ectoderm undergoes vast migrations into other anatomical sites during this embryological stage of development of the human form from its early black, melanin covered seed of life.

It is critical to note that at the first 28th hours following conception there occurs in the morula an invagination of the black dot of the morula's black ectoderm surface inward to form a tube, the neural tube. The black dot tip of this inward moving neural tube balloons out to become the brain. The tube itself becomes the spinal column. On the third day following conception the morula moves from the fallopian tube into the uterus and bonds to the wall of the uterus. It is crucial to note that the first 2 hormones produced on this the 3rd day are MSH, melanocyte stimulating hormone and, HCG, human chorionicgonadotrophin hormone.

Along the line of the neural tube there is an outer layer surrounding the neural tube, the neural crest. The neural crest is a site of many blast cells, those "immortal archetypal daughter cells" from which entire lines of other cells originate such as the haemopoeitic cells as blood cells line of white and red blood cells, gonads (spermatozoa, ovum), bone cells and especially endocrine glands , and exocrine glands that line the GI tract, urogenital tract, and respiratory tract . These vast arrays of endocrine and exocrine glands are grouped together in the broad category of the APUD cell series by virtue of the fact that they all originate from the neural crest. Moreover, they still display a marking of this vestigial origin from black ectoderm by virtue of their possessing the same decarboxylase enzyme that allows a process charge transfer of the carbon atom from an early carbon atom rich melanin ectoderm. The list of endocrine glands includes the hypothalamus, pineal, pituitary, mast cells, thyroid, parathyroid, thyrocalcitonin cells, pancreas, adrenals, and the gonads (Pearse,1969;1976).

Whereas the neural tube itself in the brain becomes the C.S.F. (cerebral spinal fluid), the ventricular system that extends into the spinal cord as the central canal is lined by the C.S.F. contracting neurons (Vigh,1975;1977;1980). In the brain stem of humans, these 12 pigmented neurons of which there is a phylogenetic range of an increasing number of 12 nucleus are pigmented only humans have all 12 pigmented, the locus coenleus bring the unique for humans. Thus there is increasing pigment upward along the neural tube. This is the I33 Tissue of Horus, Amenta nerve track of 12 sites of neuromelanin nerve tract. The amenta nerve track forms a neuromelanin covering of the 3rd ventricle.

Neurogenesis

Neurogenesis is the creation of new neurons that are added to specific regions of the brain's association cortex. Neurons are the cells of the nerve tissue with extensions running to and from them carrying and communicating information in the form of electrical impulses about the operation of the body's organ systems, especially the brain. Axons are those nerve fibers that conduct these impulses away from the body of the nerve cell, where as dendrites are those nerve fibers that transmit electrical impulses toward the nerve cell body. The vast universe of neurons and their innumerable interconnections with each other comprise the mystery of the brain. New neurons that are added in neurogenesis are involved in learning and memory (Gould, 1999; Gould, 1997). The new neurons originate in the grandular layer of the dentate gyrus from the wall of the lateral ventricles sub ventricular zone (the melanin lined old morula/gastrula ectoderm of the lateral ventricles) and then migrate downward along radial glial fibers to the L.C. modulated hippocampus,amgadyla then migrate upward as L.C. pigmented neurogenesis neurons to seed the cortical association areas of the prefrontal, post frontal, inferior temporal and parietal cortex. This course of neurogenesis occurs over the course of 21 days or 3 weeks. Neurogenesis is believed to be significantly regulated by psychosocial stressors (Gould, 1997).

Within all humans , regardless of what surface racial or ethnic identification, there exists the same brain stem that contains the same black neuromelanin nerve tract, the Amenta nerve tract with black neuromelanin. These twelve centers are the (1) locus coeruleus, (2) substantia nigra, (3) brachialis, (4) paranigralis, (5) intracapularis subcerleus, (6) nervi trigeini, (7) mesencephalasius, (8) pontis centralis orates, (9) tegmenti pedennculopontis, (10) parabrachialis, (11) medialis dorsomotor, and (12) the retroambilgualis.(Olszewki,1964; Marsden,1961; Bazelon,1968; Feinchel,1968; Forrest,1972; ;1975; Lacy,1981; 1984;;Sandyk,1991; Santamarina,1958; Vigh,1975; 1977;1980;McGinnes,1989,Lindquist,1987;King,1994) All animal life with a spinal column, the vertebrates, have varying degrees of neuromelanin pigmentation of these twelve centers. The earlier life forms such as fish, amphibians and reptiles have fewer of the twelve centers to be pigmented. Whereas the phylogenetically advanced forms have more of the centers pigmented with mammals having the largest number of neruomelanin pigmented brain melanin centers. Then within the primate family it is the near human type chimpanzee that has eleven of the twelve centers containing the most deep black neuromelanin pigmentation.

Humans are the only primate, and only vertebrate life form, to have deep neuromelanin pigmentation of the twelfth twelve-brain center. The one brain center deeply pigmented only in humans is the Locus Coeruleus. The Locus (Sanskrit/point) Coeruleus (Latin/black) means Black Dot. This 12 steps of a 12 Black nucluei is a brainstem line of neuromelanin is named the Amenta Nerve Tract. The amenta nerve track is a neuromelanin nerve tract that in humans is found in the center of the midline of the brain's spinal column that surrounds the C.S.F. (cerebral spinal fluid) ventricular system that by virtue of its morula ectoderm origin is found as a subventricular layer below the epithelium/C.S.F. containing neurons lining of the ventricular system.. It runs from the wing like lateral ventricle, especially surrounding the mid line 3rd ventricle- aqueduct of Slyvius, 4th ventricle, leading into the central canal throughout the entire spinal column. Significantly, as vertebrate life forms developed increased brain complexity there was a progressively increasing pigmentation of centers more anteriorally higher up the C.S.F. ventricle tree. It is noted that as humans have evolved from Australopithecus through to homo erectus to Homo Sapiens Sapiens, our own species, that the expansion of the cerebral cortex has witnessed increased pigmentation of the L.C. and an expansion of the cerebral cortex, neurogenesis pigmented cortical neurons.

Cells of the locus coeruleus (L.C.) provide the principal noradrenergic, norepinephrine, nerve supply to many areas of the brain-, especially the cerebral cortex, hippocampus, cingulate gyrus and amygdula areas that make up the major portion of the hippocampal limbic cortex. (Amaral.1977; Kobayshi,1975).Thus in the neurogenesis migration of new neurons from the lateral ventricle through the limbic system, it is certain that such neurons are profoundly encoded by input from the amenta nerve track/black neuromelanin nerve tract through its upper most L.C.center. There is neuromelanin charge transfer of discrete information signals conducted along the neuromelanin amenta nerve track into the migrating new neurons. This is the emotional coloring or tagging of thought, the development of much higher order neural melanin "chips" if you will. The, hard wire new neurons that are then seeded into four critical cortical association sites to expand and further uplift the thought patterns of the individual and group in its collective conscious development. In this manner, emotions at times, especially sacred or "awe inspiring times, can be signals that may expand consciousness to higher levels of expression. Similarly, the L.C. supplies part of the norepinephrine found in other brain areas such as the hypothalamus, thalamus, pineal glands, habenula (deep pineal) cerebellum; lower brain stem, and the spinal cord.

However, stress can abort neruogenesis levels leading to increased cell death of these new neurons before such neurons complete the cycle of development form a lateral ventricle birth, through limbic system modulation, followed by migration to cortical association areas. During such stress events is increased norepinephrine and uncoupling of serotonin from norepinephrine. In the normal person with a normal lower level norepinephrine increased serotonin and norepinphrine and lower levels of serotonin psychosocial stress inhibits new neuron cell proliferaton. Furthermore, "Gould reported rapid suppression of cell proliferation by a threatening experience, conveyed by cues form different sensory modalities (visual,) is a correlation of the dentate gyrus that is common to mammalian species that undergo adult neurogenesis (Gould, 1997)".

Thus, on the issue of threshold switching, there is an even larger array in the role of melanin functions as reported by Breathwatch (Breatwatch, 1988). These are the roles other than the skin or eye (Ptah, 1978, Drager, 1986) and the site of the inner ear (Meyer Zum Gottesberge, 1988). These are the neuromelanin /I33 tissue of melanin sites in the 12 pigmented nucluei of the Amenta nerve tract were neuromelanin functions in the multiple roles of threshold switch. Neuromelanin appears to provide a threshold for electrical signal conversion redox capacity, an electron transfer agent, an amorphous semiconductor threshold switch, an electron-photon couples, and also act as an accumulator of drugs and metal ions, carbon exchange properties and as a reservoir for trace elements and a sink for free species. It also acts to selectively refine energy signals from one state to another with the living neural system

A consideration of the ancient African symbolic metaphor of the all black rose granite cube shape king's chamber of the great pyramid, with open empty rose granite sarcophagus is the black inner brain chamber with each corner standing as a symbolic reference to the neuromelanin, locus coeruleus-amenta nerve endured 3rd ventricle. This dark inner brain chamber of all humans is indeed an enigma, a supreme mystery of blackness. Please consider this meager theory as prayer or mediation, as a reaching up, and a trying to understand such visions of blackness.

First in the 3rd ventricle there is a very critical linkage between the C.S.F. fluid of the 3rd ventricle that contains high concentrated levels of hormone signals from the various endocrine glands including the pineal, pituitary, gonads, urogenital gland, G.I. tract, and respiratory tree, etc. Secondly, there is a likely translation and further modulation of such signals by the C.S.F. contracting neurons that are then conveyed by the L.C. into higher thought patterns of new neurons is the association cortex. Further selective refinements of energy signals of light and gaseous liquid, lead to higher emotional, sexual, sound or auditory experience that further elevates though patterns and continues to physically charge neurons such that this high order sensing and unfoldment leads to inner vision, ascensions of the 5 senses and eventually unity with light. This all to suggest that a dormant field singularly may exist in the third ventricle that ,at a critical threshold ,allows the inner vision to undergo a 360° expansion . This Bark of Ra, in the classical Kemetic tradition of meditation, allows for the emergence of advanced sensory and intuitive experiences.

Clinical Correlations of I33 Tissue of Horus/Amenta Nerve Tract/Neuromelanin

When considering the underlying conceptual and clinical aspects of this brain stem neuromelanin operation in all humans Naim Akbar (1985) suggested that the European branch of this African root species has undergone a subtle kind of de-evolution that has 2 basic tendencies- (1) sexism or the patriarchial fear and denigration of the feminine and (2) racism, the fear and denigration of bloodline African peoples. In this context it is important to note that with many European-Africans there is indeed, clinically speaking, a legacy of pineal gland calcification which has resulted in lower levels of pineal melatonin and pineal serotonin (King, 1994). It is reported to be about ½ of the levels found in African populations. (King,1994b;Pelham,1973; Vaughn,1976). Thus with the critical differences between high skin level melanin (African-African) of the parent population and their children, European-Africans of low skin melanin, there has been a shift in the population to a lower level of melatonin. This is a critical finding of low pineal melatonin and low pineal serotonin in a European-African dominated world may go a long way in explaining the tendency of white supremacy programs that seek and continues to enforce designs that perpetuate low pineal melatonin/serotonin in themselves and their dominated African-African parents. A condition or stage of high fear of inner vision born of an aborted inherent identification with the psychological Blackness is the birth of mental slavery. In a world order dominated by the paradigm of white supremacy the white mental slave attempts to drive the fear of the psychological Blackness/conversation with one's bloodline genetic Black ancestors and the same mental slavery into others. Accordingly, in the pre-white supremacy world of Pharaoh Tutankhamen, the study of the operation of the I33 Tissue of Horus, the Amenta nerve track, was the development of inner vision through the 3 grades of students with high melataonin/serotonin, and conscious neurogenetic propagation and learning even in the face of fear. Whereas in the present white supremacy dominated world there is high norepinephrine NE, low pineal melatonin/serotonin propagation and aborted neurogenesis. It is this incomplete neurogenesis in adulthood that stops learning and keeps us worshiping the false images of the Divine in the face of fear. There is a fundamental effort embedded in the paradigm of white supremacy to enforce fear, promote images of an immense pain, misery, and castrations of Black people, all replete with a real history the lynching of people of color all the while attempting to hide the higher sciences that are born of this inner Blackness. The ediface of a fragmented material science is then used as propaganda in a dismal attempt to obscure the educational programs that the enhance development of this inner vision.

Yet, in the treatment of people in the fear based Eurocentric molds that have a high N.E. low serotonin the technique remains the same. The treatment is to review the individual and family history of the client to I.D. those symptomatic and emotionally laden trigger events and sensory experiences that are historically linked to the fear based trauma, the conditions present at the time of the trauma and the inappropriate guilt or blame assumed by the person (with results in a damaged eye of Heru). Then comes the review of that persons life and support system to find the pieces of the inspired eye, to knit the damaged lateral eye of outer vision into the awakened eye of inner vision, a dual cultural hemispheric multisensory experience of intense logical and Kemetic 'Way of the Heart' focused paths blended together by finding the Black Dot pupils ,those core creative passions given to one by the god force(Higher power) and , because of their affinity with light itself, possessed by neuromelanin modulated neurons. This is the literal Black Ben stone that is daily light infused by the Bennu bird, light itself, the soul of Ra(Higher powers). This has been from time memorial the human family's epic struggle, to locate other awakened humans, symbolized by the stories and myths of Angels-genies etc, follow their disciplines and realize the promise that some day in each one of us this power for transformation will be awakened.

Upon review of the right panel of the second shrine it appears that the upper register details a process of epigenetic enfoldment of the 3 different grades of inner vision. During the development of inner vision all 3 planes in the same person exist at the same time, but in different dimensions yet concurrently interpenetrate each other at the same moment. On the neophyte plane there is a struggle to hold onto the flesh, a belief that the material world as real, and therefore a fear of the loss of the physical body. It is the fear mentally that dreads the decay of the flesh, the physical self of creation and instrument of embodiment. In the next or high stage, the stage of Intelligence, there is the development of knowing that physical body is but a doorway through which the soul interacts with of eye of Heru, the eye of illumination, and the inner vision is awakened and moves like a river through the soul and has communication with and experiences of existence in so many other worlds. Through this doorway is housed, by the Morning Bark of Ra, the awakened spiritual consciousness, the Eye of Heru, our capacity for travel and communication with the celestial family of ancestors and spirits in the higher realms of mind and consciousness.

In summary, the operation of I33 tissue of Horus, the neuromelanin nerve tract, makes known this ancient African education system (James,1954; King,1990; Budge, 1967;Welsing,1990;Nobles,1976;Faulkner,1969;Piankoff,1977;;Clark,1975 McGee,1976,Moore,2002;Bynum,1999) promoting the progressive refinement of passionate emotional processes that results in increased melatonin/serotonin and neurogenesis of high new neuronal development even in the face of fear. The seeding of such higher order modulated emotion means that as the ascension cortex literally transforms the brain/whole body to allow an ascension of not only vision but all of the souls' capacity for unity with light and communication with what has been known since ancient times as the immortal (ancestors). This is the genius level of ideal perfections, the primordial realm of archetypal Intelligences envisioned on the banks of the Nile millennia ago. This is the union of oneself with the supreme god, traveling in the Morning Bark of Ra. "Finally, the frenzy of" Shouting" when the spirit of the lord passed by, and, seizing the devotee made him mad with supernatural joy (Holy Ghost) was the essential of Negro religion and the one believed of Negro religion and one more devoutly believed in than all the rest." (Dubois,1906) This " supernatural joy" is to travel in the many realms of the living, knowing well the full numerical symbolism and associated multilevel sensory experiences of the entire line of humanity's ancestors in light, song, and rhythmic harmony. For it is through our melanin with all its properties that African peoples and, perhaps by extension all peoples since the African genotype is the template for our species, to experience that supernatural joy, those high feeling states and come directly to experience being "touched by the spirit". It is that fleeting glimpse of our souls that is the inner vision of the genius KA, a genius and light that now reawakens (Gregory,2003).

Epilogue

ON. I give you the Eye of Heru, because of which the Gods were merciful.ON. I give you the Eye of Heru betake yourself to it. ON.,I give you the lesser Eye of Heru, of which Seth ate..ON., I give you the Eye of Heru, with which mouth is opened. The pupil which is in the Eye of Heru, eat it. ON. I give you the Eye of Heru; and you will not be ill.

Utterance 935, Coffin Texts 2100-1675 B.C.E.Kemetic Middle Kingdom (Faulkner,1978)

REFERENCES

Adams,H.H., 1994 MA'AT: Returning to Virtue-Returning to Self. Chicagi,Ill:-------

Akbar,N.,1985 Nile valley Origins of the Science of the Mind. Nile Valley Civilizations. Proceedings of the Nile Valley Conference. Atlanta,GA: Journal of African Civilizations,2,120-132

Allen, T.G. (1974) *The Book of the Dead or Going Forth by Day*, Chicago: University Chicago Press

Anders,E. and Zinner,E. 1993 Metoritcs, 28,490

Andrews,S.M.,1989 Color Me Right...Then Frame Me in Motion.Tenn; Seymore-Smith,Inc

Ani,M. 1994 Yurugu: An African-Centered Critique of European Thought and Behavior. Trenton,N.J: African World Press,Inc

Assagioli,R., 1965 Psychosynthesis : A Manual of Principles and Techniques, NY, ,N.Y: Viking Press,1-20

Astraw, B, White, T, and et al.,1999 *Australopithecus garhi: A new species of early hominid from Ethiopia*, Science, 284, 629-635

Barr,F,E., 1982 Melanin and the Mind-Body Problem. Institute for the Study of Consciousness. Berkeley:Ca

Barr,F.E., 1983 Melanin: The Organizing Molecule. Medical hypothesis,11,1-140.

Barnes,C. 1988 melanin: The Chemical Key to Black Greatness,Vol 1. Houston,TX: C.B. Publishers

Barnes,C. 1993 Jazzy Melanin: A Novel. Houston,TX: Melanin Technologies

Bazelon,M., Feinchel,G.M., 1968 Studies on neuromelanin 1: a melanin system in the human adult brainstem. Neurology,18,817-820

Ben Jochannan,Y., 1972 Black Man of the Nile and His Family, N.Y.,N.Y: Alkebu-Lan Books Associates

Bernal,M. 1991 Black Athena: The Afroasiatic Roots of Classical Civilization,Vol I: The Archaeological and Documentary Evidence. New Brunswick, N.J: Rutgers University Press

Blackshaw,S. and Snyder,S.H., 1999 Encephalopsin: a novel mammalian extraretinal opsin discretely localized in the brain, Journal of Neuroscience,19,(10), 3681-3690

Bradley,J.P. and Brownlee,D.E. 2002 Cometary Partricles: Thin sectioning and electron beam analysis. Science, 231, 1542-1544

Breathwatch, A.S., (1988); *Extra-cutaneous melanin*, Pigment Cell Research, 238-249

Brunet, M., Guy, F., et al,2002 *A New hominid from the Upper Miocene of Chad*, Central Africa, Nature, 418, p. 145-151

Bynum,E.B, (1999) The African Unconscious: Roots of Ancient Mysticism and modern Psychology, Columbia University Teachers College Press, NY

Bynum,E.B,(1994) Transcending Psychoneurotic Disturbances: New Approaches in Psychospirituality and Personality Development,NY, Haworth Press

Bynum,E.B. 1984 The Family Unconscious: An Invisible Bond. Wheaton,Ill: Theosophical Publishing House

Budge,E.A.W., 1969 The God of The Egyptians, V. 1 & 2, N.Y: Dover Publications

Budge,E.A.W., 1923 Tutankhamen,Amenism, Atenism and Egyptian Monotheism. N.Y.,N.Y: Dell Publishing Company

Budge., W.E.A., 1967 The Book Of the Dead. N.Y.,N.Y: Dover Publication

Clark,X.,C., McGee,P.P.,Nobles,W., 1975 Voodoo or I.Q.: An introduction to African Psychology. Journal of black Psychology, 1,2, 9-19

Clarke, J.H.,1999 My Life In Search of Africa, Chicago,Ill: Third World Press

Chruchward,A., 1921 The Origin and Evolution of the Human Race, London: George-Allen and Unwin,Ltd

Churchward, A. (1924) *The Origin and Evolution of Religion*, N.Y.,N.Y:E.P. Dutton and Company

Chruchward,A.,(1913) 1986 The Signs and Symbols of Primordial man.Evolution of Religious Doctrines from the Eshatology of the Ancient Egyptians. London: Second edition,George Allen& Company.Ltd, N.Y:,E.P.Dutton & Company

Cotzias, G.C., Papa Vasiliou P.S., Van Woort M.H., Sakamoto, A; 1964 Fed. Proc. 23, 713

Diop,C.A. 1981 Origin of the Ancient Egyptians, General history of Africa,,Vol.11., ancient Civilizations of Africa,G.Mokhtar ed, Berkeley,CA: University of California Press

Diop, C.A. (1991), *Civilization or Barbarism*, West Port, CN: Lawrence Hill & Co.

Drager, U.C., (1986) *Albinism and Visual Pathways*, The New England Journal of Medicine V. 314, 25, 636

Dubois,W.E.B. 1906 The Souls of Black Folk, New york,N.Y:Bantam Books

Falk, D. ,Redmond, J G., et.al,1999 *Early hominid brain evolution: A new look at old endocrasts*, Journal of Human Evolution, 38, 695-717

Faulkner,R.O.,1969 The Ancient Egyptian Pyramid Texts, . Oak Park,Ill:Aris and Phillips,Ltd Bolchazy-Carducci

Faulkner,R.O., 1978 The Egyptian Coffin texts.v1-111,England: Westminster

Feinchel,G.M. 1968 Studies on neuromelanin 2: melanin in the brainstem of infants and children. Neurology,18, 817-820

Forrest,F.M. 1975 The evolutionary role of neuromelanin. West Pharmacol. ,18,205

Gould, E., McEwin, B.S., Tanapat, P., Glen, L.A.M., Fushs, E. 1997 *Neurogenesis in the dentate gyrus of the adult tress shrew is regulated by psychosocial stress and NMDA receptor activation*, Journal of Neuroscience, 17 (7) 2492-2498, 1997

Guderian,H.,Panzer Leader,P.D.A., 1952 Cambridge ,MA: Kopo Press

Gould, E., Reeves, A.J., Grazians, L.A., Gross, G.G.;1999 *Neurogenesis in the neocortex of adult primates*, Science, 286,548-552

Gould,E. 1999 Serotonin and hippocampal neurogenesis, Neuropsychopharmacology, 21; 463-515

Gould,E., McEwen,B.S., Tanapat,P.,Galea,L.A.M., Fuch,S.E. 1997 Neurogenesis in the dentate gyrus of the adult Tressshrew regularius by psychosocial stress and NMDA receptor activation. The Journal of Neuroscience, 17(7), 2492-2498

Gregory,D,2003 The Legacy of Dr. Martin Luther King,Something Greater than Fear or
Hatred. Black Psychiatrists of America, Section V of the National Medical Association, Beverly Hills,Ca

Hill, H.G.M., Jones,K.P., and d'Hendecourt, 1998 Diamonds in carbon-rich proto-planetary nebulae. Letter to the editor, Astronomy and Astrophysics,L41-L44

Hill ., H.G.M., Jones, A.P., and d'Hendecourt,L.B. 1998 Letter to the editor, Astronomy and Astrophysics, 336, L41-L44

Howe,S. 1998 Afrocentrism: Mythical Pasts and Imagined Homes,N.Y: Verso

Jablonski, N.G., Chaplin, G.T.2000, The evolution of human coloration. *Journal of Human Evolution*. 39, 57-106

Jackson, J.G. (1970) *Introduction to African Civilizations*, New York, University Books
James, G.G.M. (1954) *Stolen Legacy*, New York, Philosophical Library
Janata, P., Birk, J.L., Van Horn, J.P., Leman, M., Tillmannn, B., Bharucha, J.J., (2002), *The Cortical Topography of Tonal Structures Underlying Western Music*, Science, 298, 2167-2270.
Jantsch,E 1980 The Self-Organizing Universe. N.Y,N.Y: Pergamon Press
Jorgenson,V.G., 1988 nature,322,702
Kappelman, J, Swisher IV, C C., et al,1996 *Age of Austrolopitheus Africans from Fejej*, Ethiopia, J. of Human Evolution, 30, 139-146
Kershaw,I., 1998 Hitler 1889-1936 Hubris, N.Y.,N.Y: W.W. Norton Co
Kershaw,I., 1999, Hitler, 1937-1945 Nemesis, N.Y.,N.Y: W.W.Norton
Kimbel; W, H., Johnson, D, C., et al,1994 *The First Skull and other new discoveries of Austratopitheus Afarensic at Hada*, Ethiopia, Nature, 308
King,R.D.,(1990) The African Origin of Biological Psychiatry. Chicago,Ill: Lushena Books
King,R.D. 1992 Kemetic Images of Light,Sunlight and Moon Light Durhan,N.C.King,R.D., 1993 Black symbolism of the unconscious: Part 1,Review of Black symbolism in the collected works(v1-20) of C.G.Jung,1933
King,R.D., 1994b The pineal gland , melanin and calcium: pineal gland calcification in African=Americans, a review of 1,622 cases; a scientific essay. N.C:Durham
King,R.D. 1994 Melanin: The Key to Freedom, Chicago,Ill: Lushena Books
Kobayashi,R., 1975 Biochemical mapping of the noradrenergic projection from the locus coeruleus. Neurology
Kume,K.Siram,S.,Shearman,L.P., Weaver,D.R., Jin,X., Maywood,E.S., Hastings,M.H. and Reppert,S.M., 1999, MCRY and MCRYZ are essential components of the negative limb of clock feedback loop. Cell. 193-205
Lacy,M. 1981 Neuromelanin: a hypothetical component of bioelectric mechanisms in brain function. Physiol. Chem. & Physics,13,319-324
Lacy,M. 1984 Phonon-electron coupling as a possible transducing mechanism in bioelectronic processes involving neuromelanin. Journal of Theoretical Biology,111, 201-204
Leakey, G.,1995 *New four-million-year-old hominid species from Ranapoi and Allia Bay*, Kenya, Nature 376, 565-571
Leigh, S H.,1992 *Cranial Capacity Evolution in HomoErecteus and Early Homosapiens*, American Journal of Physical Anthropology, 87; 1-13
Lewis,R.S., Anders,E., and Draine,B.T. 1989 Nature,339,117

Luu,J.X., 1993 Spectral diversity among the nuclei of comets. Icarus,104
Liou, J.C., Zook, H.A. and Dermott, S.F. 1996 Kuiper Belt dust grains as a source of interplanetary dust particles,Icarus,124, 429-440
Lindquest,N.G., 1987 Neuromelanin and its possible protective and destructive properties. Pigment cell Research,!:133-136
Lindquist, N.G.1973, Acta Radiol- 325
Marsden,C.D. 1961 Pigmentation in the nucleus substantia nigra in primates. Journal of Comparative Anatomy
McGee,P. 1976 An Introduction to African Science: Melanin, the physiological basis for psychological oneness, in L.M.King et al (eds) African Philosophy: Assumptions and Paradigms For Research On Black Persons. Los Angeles,CA: Fanon Center Publications
McGinness, J., Corry, P., Proctor, P. (1974), *Amorphous semiconductor switching in melanins*, Science, 853-855
McGinness,J.E., 1985 A new view of pigmented neurons. Journal of Theoretical Biology,115,475-476
McGinness,J., Corry,P.,Proctor,P. 1974 Science, 183, 853-855
McHenry, H,, Berger,M Lee R., 1998 *Body proportions in Austraopithecus*, Journal of Human Evolution, 35, 1-22
Calif,N.M.A.:past ancestors, my immediate family, my extended family and my future ancestors.
Moore,T.O. 1995 The Science of Melanin,Dispelling The Myths Silver Spring,M.D.: Venture Books,Beckham House Publishers
Moore,T.O., 2002 dark Matters, Dark Secrets. Redan,GA: Zamani Press
Moore,R.Y., Speh,J.C., and Card,S.P. 1995 The retinohypothalmic tract originates from a distinct subset of retinal ganglion cells. Journal of Comparative Neurology, 352, 351-366
Nicolas,B.R.J., Nicolas, R.A., 1998 Biological garbage or jewels. Scientific communication presented at the meeting of the European Society for Pigment Cell Research. Sept 23-26(1998), Prague, Pigment Cell Research,11, 233
Nicolas,R.A., 1997 Colored organic semiconductors: melanins rend, Acc. Sc. Fis. Mat. Napolis, vol. LXIV, 325-360
Nicolas,B.R.J., and Nicolas,R.A. 1997 Speculating on the band colors in nature, Atti dell Accademia. pontananiana, Giannini, Napoli, vol. XLV,365
Nobles,W. 1986 African Psychology: Toward Its Reclaimation, Reascension and Revitalization. Oakland,CA: A Black family Institute Publication
Nobles, W. 1976 African Science and Black Research,The Consciousness of Self, in L.King,V.Dixon and W. Nobles(eds) African Philosophy: Assumptions

and Paradigms for Research on Black People. Los Angeles,CA: Fanon Research and Development Center Publications
Nuth,J.A.,Allen,J.D.E. 1992 Astrophysics and Space Science,196,117
Olswezski,J. 1964 Cytoarchitecture of the Human Brain Stem. N.Y: Sternnam Birjelow
Path, M.O., (1978) *Phagocytes of Light and Dark Adapted Rod Outer Segments by Cultural Epithelium*, Science, 203, 526
Pearse,A.G.E., 1969 The cytochemical ultra structure of cells of the APUD series and the embryologic physiologic implications of the concept . Journal of Histochemistry and Cytochemistry, 17(5), 303-313
Pearse,A.G.E., 1976 Neuroendocrine embryology and the APUD concept. Clinical Endocrinology, S. Supplement,2335
Pelham,W. Vaughn,G., Sandock,K., Vaughn,M. 1973 Twenty-four hour cycle of a melatonin-like substance in the plasma of human males. Journal of Clinical Endocrinology Metalo. 37,341-344
Petrie,W. 1939 The Making of Egypt. London: Fig.1,p 86-89
Piankoff,A., 1954 The Tomb of Ramses VI , Bollingen Series,XL-I, N.Y: Pantheon Books,208
Piankoff,A. 1977 The Shrines of Tutankhamen, Bollingen SeriesXL, Princeton,N.J; Princeton University Press
Pickard, G.E. 1982 . The afferent connections of the suprachiasmatic nucleus of the golden hamerster with emphasis on the retinohypothalmic projection. Journal of Comparative Neurology,211,65-83
Pandey,S., Blanks,J.C., Spee,C.,Jiang,M. and Fong,H.F.W., 1994 Cytoplasmic retinal localization of an evolutionary homolog of the visual pigments. Experimental Eye Research,58,605-613
Proctor, P.1972; Physical Chem. Phys. 4, 349
Reed, K.. E.;1997 *Early hominid evolution and ecological change through the African pilo-pleistocence,* Journal of Human Evolution, 32, 289-322
Santamarina,E 1958 Melanin pigmentation in bovine pineal gland and its possible correlation with gonadal function. Journal of biochem. Physiol., 36,227-335
Sandyk,R. 1999 Relavance of the habenular complex to neuropsychiatry: a review and hypothesis. International Journal of Neuroscience, 61,189-219
Skelton,R.R., and McHenry,H.H., 1992 Evolutionary relationships among early hominids, Journal of Human Evolution, 23,309-349
Tielens,A.G.G., Seab,C.G., and Hollenback,D.J. Abj,319,L109
Tobias, P, V.,1987 *The bones of homohahilia: A new level of organization in cerebral evolution.* J of Human Evolution, 16, 741-761

Van Kerekhoven,C., Tielens,A.G.G.M., and Waelkens,C., 2002 Nanodiamonds around HD 9704B and Elias 1. Astronomy and Astrophysics 384, 568-584

Vaughan,G., Pelham,R., Pang,R., Loughlin,L. Wilson,K. Sandock,K.,Vaughan,M. Koslow,S. Reiter,R. 1976 Nocturnal evaluation of plasma melatonin and urinary S-hydroxyindolencetic acid in young men: attempts at modification by brief changes in enviormmental lighting and sleep by autonomic drugs. Journal of clinical Endocrinology Metab. 42, 752-764

Vigh,B. 1975 Comparative ultra structure of cerebrospiunal fluid contacting neurons and pinealocytes. Cell Tissue Research, 158,409-424

Vigh,B., 1977 Special dendritic and axonal endings formed by the cerebrospinal fluid contacting neurons of the spinal cord. Cell Tissue Research, 183, 541-552

Vigh-Teichmann,I. 1980 Comparison of the pineal complex and cerebrospinal fluid contacting neurons by immunl cytochemical antirhodopsin Mikokanat. Fuesch. Leipzig. 94,:4(8), 623-640

Welsing,F.C., 1990 The Isis Papers: Keys to the Colors. Chicago,Ill: Third World Press

Webster's Dictionary

West,J.A. 1993 Serpent In The Sky: The High Wisdom of Ancient Egypt.Wheaton,Ill:Theosophical Publishing House

Wimby-Jones,R.A. 1982 Private communication.Commentary and the translation of the right panel of the second shine from the tomb of pharaoh Tutankhamen,.The Kemetic Institute,Chicago,Ill

Wood, B.,2000 Review, *Human evolution: taxonomy and paleobiology,* Journal of Anatomy 196, p. 19-60

Zatorre, R.J. & Kruahansi, C.L. (2002) Mental Models and Musical Minds, Science, 298,2138-2139

Thank you for the fabulous support of the Council of Elders to the Km Wr,Inc, and to Dr.John Henrik Clark and Dr. Yusef ben Jochannan; Eye of Heru study group of Detroit,Aquarian Spiritual Center of Los Angeles:First World of New York: ASCAC, Dept of Black Studies, San Francisco State University: Fanon R & D Center, N.1.M.H.: Black Psychiatrists of America.

POSTSCRIPT

Data is not knowledge and knowledge is not wisdom but when ancient wisdom is married to new knowledge it may suggest a radically transcendent vision of reality. From the introduction we sought to place this study within the context of humankind's ongoing scientific exploration of itself and its place in the cosmos. The more our species has explored the world within itself, the more it has seen itself reflected in the world outside.. "As above, so below, as within, so without", the principal revelation of Tehuti and the core of the hermetic corpus of ancient writings became the root metaphor of a scientific and spiritual intuition that in Ages that followed has given birth to innumerable discoveries, inventions and intimate understandings of ourselves. Like mathematics it yokes us to the world process and its most luminous permutations.

Beginning in the first chapter with Professor Moore we tried to harness the new knowledge of embryogenesis or life and development in the womb to focus on how evolution's drama of increasing complexity was intimately involved in the dynamics of melanin and neuromelamim. Melanin's capacity to interact with light and transmute it to higher levels of order and complexity, to transform it from one state of energy to another, was seen as a crucial parallel to evolution itself. Indeed melanin and neuromelanin in particular was no longer seen as a mere biochemical "waste product" of the nervour system but rather an intimate player in the drama of life's mysterious unfoldment into more rarified expressions of intelligence and light.The fact that neuromelanin appears to absorb light and to increase indensity and amount as we progress or "ascend" up the evolutionary ladder only deepened this sense of an intimate embrace with the dance of evolution.

This was particularily important when we saw how, given its unique properties as an energy transducer, neuromelanin facilitated nerve conduction in the cerebral structures. This is not limited to the transfer of charge over the surface of the neuron, but crucially *between* neurons in the snaptic space where electrochemical transduction occurs. It is this "gap" or space between snaptic junctures where energy and consciousness itself seem to meet we believe and establish their nonlocal romance. This is also the place where psychiatric medications have their pstchotropic influence on consciousness.

We say that energy and consciousness meet in their nonlocal romance in this space or "gap" because this space is not merely biochemical, but also molecular, and then elemental and the atomic and quantum and eventually sub-quantum and therby nonlocal in its dynamics. It is, we suggest, the place where consciousness itself unfolds out into matter from its enfolded orders.

But melanin was not restricted to the brain or even the human or mammalian body. Professor Brown's chapter elaborated on the different types of melanins found in the wider environment, including the soil, the water, the air, indeed in the wider solar system itself. The startling fact that it is also localized in strategic locations within the inner most recesses of the brain only reinforced the sense of importance of this neglected area of science. Perhaps it is because melanins are found from the reaches of the solar system to the inner sanctum of the brain core, that the widest "outer" in some physical and energetic sense reflects the deepest "inner", denies us a clear boundary between these realms and is a confession that in some still mysterious way they reflect each other. Science can never be completely divorced from metaphysics any more than energy can be from information and yet the two are not identical.

In our search for the meaning of life and our place amid the stars we as a species have turned our attention to the seat of our own consciousness, the brain. Like neuroanatomy itself in the early days of Kemetic Egyptian exploration of the body in the process of mummification and battlefielf trauma medicine much was discovered about mental functioning mental functioning based on neuroanatomical structures. Melanin and neuromelanin exploration in neuroscience has furthered this understanding by noting in all human beings regardless of surface so called 'racial diversification' the strategic location of neuromelanin in these brain structures, especially beyond the surface cerebral and into the deeper limbic and other sub cortical structures. By adding to it the influence and interaction of biochemistry and evolutionary neurobiology to the dynamics of light the study of neurmelanin has implicated the subtle loom of consciousness itself. It has an affinity to light. Light remains our most fundamental mirror and intuition of matter itself.

By the mid point of this book we turned our attention to consciousness itself and its involvement with neuromelanin. Beyond the medical and physical involvement of neuromelanin with stress symptoms of psychosomatic disorders it was emphasized how the many mid brain limbic system of neuromelanin foci interacted with higher cerebral structures in the modulation of emotions, feelings, images and memories. Emotionally powerful symbolic images were seen as particularly evocative.

Essentially we suggested that in a very real way we *consciously interact with neuromelanin* through our emotional and somatic experiences. This includes not only our personally informed memories and experiences, but also our socially informed collective and deeper contemplative experiences born of our psychospiritual disciplines stretching back millennia through innumerable traditions from all branches of our species. Realization in the contemplative disciplines leads to the dissolution of all experiential categories of internal and external space and opens into a luminous confluence of self, other and numinous processes in which space, time, matter and location are derivative notions ofa deeper , more enfolded order. This was true in antediluvian Kemet on the banks of the Nile before the raising of the pyramids as it was in ancient Tibet on down to the refined meditative disciplines of the post modern age. Neuromelanin with its affinity to light and consciousness is an intimate aspect of our nature despite the seeming differences in our external appearance and is here reemerging into the context of contemporary science.

Tehuti,Hermes Tresmigistis, the inward systems of order in flowing permutation with the wider outside cycles of the cosmos, this is the ancient vision coming to rebirth in our times. Nowhere is this more in evidence that when Dr. King explores the stellar dynamics of the solar expanse and the intimate process of the neural net. It is Dr. King along with Dr. Moore who drew our clinical attention to neurogenesis or the evolution of new neural cells and Dr. King who drew this connection to cosmology or the solar expanse.

Neurocosmology is as old as the human mind itself and rooted in the same soil as our collective progenitors in Africa. It is indeed an irony of the current Age that with this being rediscovered the very peoples who initially discovered and formulated this principal of the world process, the peoples of northeast and west Africa, should find themselves in the economic and geopolitical fix that they do today.

There have been many rises, many falls, many forgotten triumps and resurrections of the peoples of Africa. But how could it not be so, for Africa is the genetic and anthropological root of the human species with all its permutations and dramas and the deep brain core carries this primordial narrative through all its variations in the diverse peoples of the earth. Today, despite the daily drumbeat of negative news about poverty, disease, war, malnutrition, corruption, indeed every plague known to humanity attacking the continent and its people, Africa is again slowly ascendant. In recent centuries the fall of Africa again, after another cyclical rise during its medieval ages, lead to an unprecendented spread of African slavery and degradation. Dark skin, especially in the European dominated world, became identified with a fallen state and took on near mythical porportions, spreading its racially infected ideology into the tacit assumptions of science, religion, politics, and even into the intimate dynamics of social and family life. Dark skin became a sign of a lessened status, a fractional membership in the human family. The very study of anything dark skinned or *even associated with dark skin* became taboo or else feared, denigrated and devalued.

A similar history occurred in Dravidian India when the indo Aryans swept down from the north and through war executed over a hundred years essentially enslaved the dark skinned inhabitants of the Indus valley. The British episode reinforced this notion.

It is a curious irony that in both narratives the dark skinned inhabitants had created and nurtured, centuries before the invaders, highly disciplined contemplative sciences that sought to raise and fill the inner sanctum of the human mind with a luminous reality that connected it with the stars and a reality beyond linguistic conceptualization. In the Indus valley it was called yoga, in Kemet it was a similar science. The Indo Aryans took the science to themselves and over time, in a process of **cryptoamnesia**, *forgot its origins* in the conquered low caste dark skinned peoples they came to despise. Early Islam, Christianity and Judiasm all have their historical roots in the soil of dark skinned peoples. This is no coincidence. It was no accident either that these two subjugated civilizations for thousands of years before their conquest were in contact with each other through the land and sea lane trade routes of the Indian ocean. What is crucial for our study here is that in both cases they discovered how to awaken and illuminate the inner darkness of every human mind with a kind of living bio-light that was an intimate part of the body, the brain and the deep brain core. That brain core vibratory reality we suggest here is an actived and awakened neuromelanin nerve tract.

In the post modern Age identity politics is all to real. The taboo of embracing our collective dark skinned African origins living in our very brain is ironically similar to the taboo that prevents us from embracing the paradoxically dark luminosity thuis brain core and its surface confesses about who we really are and where we all come from regardless of our mere surface appearances. Both in many cases leads to the dissolution of a more dominant politically, culturally and even psycho religiously informed sense of self while offering instead an uncharted, boundless and terrifyingly radiant state of consciousness.

In the modern 'Western world' people often want "a healthy tan" but also the perks of white privilege. People want to be religious but generally are afraid of having a religious experience. Therein lies our postmodern dilemma and we are all dimlyaware of it. We just don't quite know what to do about it either.

We are suggesting here that the study of melanin and neuromelanin may just offer us a way to collectively heal ourselves and transcend this dilemma. Melanin on the skin's surface in recent centuries in large areas of the world has tended to be used to divide us, dehumanize us, teach us to marginalize our humanity and contract our collective sense of an interwoven identity. Now neuromelanin, anlagen of our shared origins, an echo of our collective identity rooted in the nerve work itself, suggests a pathway out of our spiraling nightmare of hate, recoil and rampages of revenge.

It is one of the living realities that unites us in a deep place and connects us through time and differentiation with all the higher life forms of this earth. It has been there since the beginning and in a real sense been part of the conductivity of our life force as we have ascended upward through the evolutionary arch. It has quickened our nervous system activity, deepened our consciousness and made more subtle our apprehension of the seen and unseen world. No it is not the sole axis of human development. Rather it is one of the fathomless currents that flow through the oceanic mystery of who and what we are.

Someday our future science will turn its attention to what occurs vibrationally when, through discipline and techniques, the internal constellations of neuromelanin enters into a conscious *resonate affinity* with the solar ambience of melanin particles distributed throughout the solar expanse. Everything is luminous and alive moving through transformations and translations. When our ancient insight that we are luminous beings is realized then our new knowledge based on science and technology will emerge onto a vast new plane of experience. At that time when collectively we understand as a species that when 'the eye is single and the body is full of light', our progeny spread out and living on the shores of distant worlds from earth will realize the vision worked out on the banks of the Nile dateless millennia ago.
>

GLOSSARY

WHY DARKNESS MATTERS (New and Improved)

Glossary of technical terms used here and in related readings
<UNL>
Afferent: Nervous system structures that conduct fluid or nerve impulses toward an organ or other structures, e.g., afferent neurons conduct impulses to the central nervous system.

Ajna: The sixth or brow chakra located between the eyebrows.
Amenta nerve track. The melinated nerve track extending from the brainstem to the midbrain.

Anahata: The fourth or heart chakra located behind the sternum.
Apana vayu: The energy in the pelvic region; excretion, downward flow.

Asana: A physical posture of hatha yoga; the third aspect of raja yoga.

Australopithecines: Any of several extinct bipedal pre-Homo primate ancestors from millions of years ago. They are known primarily from the Pleistocene fossil period in southern and southeast Africa.

Avian system: Studies or other reseach having to do or associated with bird and birdlike systems.

Ayurveda: The medical system of the Vedas, a holistic spiritual approach.

Bandha: A contraction of part of the body designed to contain energy flow.

Bhakti yoga: The path of devotion and surrender to the divine.
Blood-brain barrier: A system of barriers (membranes, etc.) that inhabit the passage of certain molecules from the blood into brain tissue and cerebrospinal fluid.

Brahma nadi: The innermost nadi of Mehru Dandah; ends in Brahma Randhram.

Catecholamine: Any of a group of amines, which includes epinephrine, norepinephrine and dopamine, that are derived from tyrosine and have a hormonal function.

Chakra: A matrix of subtle energy vortexes in the body; six are major.

Cell culture: The growing of cells in vitro(glass), including the culture of single cells. In cell cultures, the cells are not organized into tissues (tissue cultures).

Citrini nadi: The second-subtlest nadi of Mehru Dandah; stairway route.

Complete rising: Enlightenment, a rising to the top of the crown lotus.

Cytosol (perikaryon): The cytoplasm around the nucleus in the cell body of a nerve cell. This is the liquid portion of the cell, in which is suspended other internal cell structures.

Dark Matter: The unseen so-called "cold dark matter" that is believed to account for about 93 percent of the matter in the known cosmos as presently calculated by science. It is detected by gravitational measures but its nature is currently unknown.

Deafferentation: The decrease in neural impulses or input to a specific region of the brain or nervous system, which results in a change in the usual unction of that area and its parallel psychological process.

Efferent: Pertains to those structures that lead away from organs or structures such as the efferent arteriole of the kidney nephron.

Eumelanin: The most common biological melanin, a brown-black polymer, an excellent photo protectant.

Full rising: A rising from the top of the brow to the crown lotus.

Genius: The genie or developing angel, the second stage of psychospiritual human development in the Kemetic mystery school sysyem. The second stage of development unifies both the left cortical "masculine" logical consciousness and the right cortical "feminine" emotional consciousness to

produce a unified consciousness, with an expansion and elevation of passion, logic, elevated neurogenesis, and creativity.
Granthi: Knots of nadis at three chakras blocking Saraswati nadi.

Guru: An enlightened being authorized to guide and initiate disciples.

Hatha yoga: The foundation of raja yoga; ethics, postures, breathing.

Histological Study: A microscopic study of the minute structures of cells, tissues,etc., in relation to their functions. Nerve cells are studied using a preparation under a microscope.
Horus or Heru: The ancient Kemetic Egyptian god of the sun and light as represented by the hawk-headed figure. Often associated with the life force ascending beyond death and associated with the sons/daughters of light. That third eye state of human development that results from conscious unity with the ancestral realm and the perfect fulfillment of one's core creative passion, mission and purpose for being.

Ida nadi: Nadi or energy pathway to the left of Sushumna; moon, receptive, parasympathetic.
Intermediate rising: A rising between the top of the heart and top of brow chakras.

Jnana yoga: The path of intellect involving study, contemplation, meditation.

Karma yoga: The path of loving, selfless service to the divine.
Kemet: Name often given for the 'land of the Blacks' and black soil of ancient Egypt.

Kemetic: Indigenous African people(s) of Nubia and the Ethiopian highlands who migrated down the Nile and gave rise to Egyptian civilization.

Koshas: The five sheaths; physical body, energy, mind, wisdom, bliss.

Kriya: A movement of the body caused by kundalini process.
Kundalini: The spiritual capacity or presence in a person; static or dynamic.

Kundalini arousal: The uncoiling or unblocking of kundalini in the root chakra.
Kundalini process: The activity and experiences of a kundalini rising.

Kundalini release: The initial surging forth of kundalini from the root chakra.

Kundalini rising: The upward movement of level of the released kundalini.

Kundalini yoga: The comprehensive science of raising and guiding kundalini.

Laya yoga: The yoga of dissolution; the tattvas absorbed into their subtlest.
Left path: The moderate use of sex by loving, committed couples.

Linga: A column in the root, heart, or brow chakra blocking Sushumna

Manipura: The third or navel chakra, located at the solar plexus.

Mantra: A sacred phoneme used for the effects of its vibrational properties.

Mehru Dandah: The four concentric spinal nadis; Sushumna, Vajra, Citrini, Brahma.

Melanin: A natural dark pigmentation found inside and outside the human body.Because it is dark it absorbs light.

Melanocytes. Pigment-forming cells which are predominately derived from the neural crest during early embryogenesis.

Morula: The spherical embryonic mass of blastomeres formed before complete blastulation.

Muladhara: Base or root of the spine in the yoga systems; the place of the mulabandha or root lock for kundalini energy.

Myelin Sheath: A fatty sheath-like covering of the axons of some nerve fibers. Nerve fibers that possess myelin sheaths are called myelinated nerve fibers, and those that do not are called unmyelinated nerve fibers. The myelin sheath protects the nerve fiber and transports impulses rapidly.

Nadi: An energy current within the subtle body

Neural Crest: An area bordering the neural tube that forms as an invagination of the ectoderm layer, from which cells migrate and later become specialized into melanocytes, ganglia, and many other body structures.

Neural Tube: A tube formed from the neuroectoderm of the early embryo by the closure of the neural groove; it develops into the spinal cord and brain.

Neurocosmology: The study of the subtle interrationships between the brain and the cosmos as expressed in a metaphor, symbolism, and physical and /or energetic principles and correspondences.

Neuromelanin: Photoactive and psychoactive melanin found in the brain and nervous system of the higher animals, mammals and primates, which increases as evolution becomes more complex.

Neuromelanin I33 Tissue of Heru: The black Ben-Stone of neural tissue in the brain and spinal column that transforms the experiences of living biological systems from the lower animals to the higher, then to the human, higher human, and eventually to the transcendent realms of experience and expression.

Neuron: Any of the cells of nerve tissue, consisting of a nucleated portion and cytoplastic extension.

Nigrostriatal tract: The bundle of dark nerve fibers in the brain extending from the substantia nigra to the globus pallidus and putamen in the corpus striatum, injury or degeneration to which leads to Parkinson's and other disorders.

Partial rising: A rising no higher than the top of the heart chakra.

Parietal Lobe: One of the four major sections or lobes of both hemespheres of the brain. It is interconnected with all other brain areas and is associated with sensory orientation and motor functions along with other neural processes. The other lobes are the frontal, occipital, and temporal lobes.

Between the cerebral cortex and the brainstem, within the brain itself, is another lobe, often referred to as the limbic lobe, through which information and emotional impulses flow.

Phylogenetic: The evolutionary development of animal and plant species. Their historical, structural and cultural development.
Pingala nadi: To the right of Sushumna; sun, active, sympathetic nervous system.

Pluripotent Stem Cells: Usually refers to progenitors of blood cells. Cells from the neural crest that have the potential to become many different cell types upon their differentiation.

Prana: The vital energy force in a human being; the second kosha.

Pranayama: A breathing practice that directs the flow of prana.

Quantum Mechanics: A branch of physics that deals with the extremely small shifting energy fields, matrices and sub-atomic particles that operates at or below the level of molecules and atoms. It is the microcosmic world of energy, information and vibration.

Raja yoga: Eight-limbed yoga described in Patanjali's *Yoga Sutras*.

Right path: The ascetic rechanneling of all sexual expression.
Sahasrara: The thousand-petaled lotus at the crown of the head, the seventh chakra.

Samskara: A latent impression or characteristic in the unconscious mind.

Sankhini nadi: The stem and pericarp of sahasrara from anus to lower brain.

Saraswati nadi: A nadi outside the spine on the left side, from root to brow.

Sat chit ananda: Pure unitary consciousness; knowledge-beingness-bliss.

Semiconductor: A substance that is capable of carrying energy as an efficient rapid flow of electrons.

Shakti: Divine grace; kundalini; feminine creative principle of the universe.

Shaktipat: Initiation of grace by an enlightened adept or God.
Shiva: Pure consciousness; the masculine principle of the universe.

Siddha: An adept; an enlightened being elevated to an exalted status.

Siddha yoga: Yoga of the adepts, who initiate through shaktipat.
Supraluminal: Energy and phenomena that move above light speed.

Superconscious: The realm of conscious that is above and subsumes the unconscious, preconscious and the ego.

Superconductivity: The flow of electrical current without the usual resistance of most metals, alloys and other substances; usually occurs at very low temperatures but also perhaps at room temperature in biological systems.

Sushumna: The outermost nadi of Mehru Dandah growing through the spine.

Svadhisthana: The second or genital chakra located at the prostate or uterus.

Swara: A yoga based on the science of breathing.

Tantras : Texts describing yogic practices and their results.

Tutankhamen: The young pharaoh of the 18th dynasty who returned ancient Kemetic Egypt to the worship of Amon after the fall of the worship of sun disk god Aton and restored the capital to Thebes. His wealthy royal tomb was found intact in the Valley of the Kings by Howard Carter in 1922.

Upanishad: The last part of the Veda upon which Vedanta is based.

Ureaus. The Kemetic Egyptian symbol for the serpentine energy form extending from the base of spinal line, through the brainstem into the brain core associated with the kundalini phenomenon.

Vajra nadi: The third-subtlest nadi of Mehru Dandah; sex path.
Vedas: The most ancient scriptures of Indian philosophy.
Vedanta: The philosophy based on the Upanishads, the final Vedic texts.

Vertebrate: Animals having a backbone or spinal column. Included are the fish, amphibians, reptiles, birds, mammals and man.

Vishuddha: The fifth or throat chakra located in the pit of the throat.

Yoga: A practical, dualistic philosophy with spiritual practices.

Yoga Sutras: The aphorisms of Patanjali that describe raja yoga.
Zygote: The fertilized egg cell before cleavage, created when sperm

WHY DARKNESS MATTERS Selected Further Readings

Akbar, NA'im. *Light from Ancient Africa.* Tallahassee, Fla.: Mind Productions and Associates, Inc., 1994.

Ashby, Muata A. *Egyptian Yoga: The Supreme Wisdom of Enlightenment.* Miami, Fla.: Sema Institute of Yoga, 2000.

Ashby, Muata A. *The Egyptian Book of the Dead: The Book of the Coming Forth by Day.*
    Miami, Fla.: Sema Institute of Yoga, 2000.

Ashby, Muata A. The Serpent Power: The Ancient Egyptian Mystical Wisdom of the   Inner Life Force. Miami, Fla.: Sema Institute of Yoga, 2000.

Basham, Arthur L. *The Wonder that was India.* New York City, N.Y.: Grove

Press, 1959.

Browder, Anthony T. *Egypt on the Potomac: A Guide to Decoding Egyptian Architecture and Symbolism in Washington, D.C.* Washington, D.C.: IKG Publishing, 2004.

Bender, Andrew L. "A Hypothesis for a Membrane Theory of Gravity." <http://www.BraneBrain.com> accessed 2006.

Bauval, Robert and Brophy, Thomas. *Black Genesis: The Prehistoric Origins of Ancient Egypt.* Rochester, Vt.: Inner Traditions and Bear Company, 2011.

Bauval, Robert and Hancock, Graham. *Message of the Sphinx.* New York City, N.Y.: Three Rivers Press, Crown Publishing, 1997.

Brophy, Thomas. *The Origin Map: Discovery of a Prehistoric Megalithic Astrophysical Map of the Universe.* Bloomington, Ind.: i Universe, 2002.

Bynum, Edward B. *The Roots of Transcendence.* New York City, N.Y.:Cosimo Books.2003. Formally titled *Transcending Psychoneurotic Disturbances.* Haworth Books, 1994.

Bohm, David. *Wholeness and the Implicate Order.* London, UK.: Routledge and Kegan Paul, 1980.

Bohm, David. *Causality and Chance in Modern Physics* (1957). Harper 1961 edition reprinted in 1980. Philadelphia. Pa.: University of Pennsylvania Press.

Halpern, Paul. *The Great Beyond: Higher Dimensions, Parallel Universes and the Extraordinary Search for a Theory of Everything.* Hoboken, N.J.: John Wiley and Sons, 2004.

Krauss, Lawrence M. *Hiding in the Mirror: The Mysterious Allure of Extra Dimensions, from Plato to String Theory and Beyond.* New York City, N.Y.: Viking Books, 2005.

Gates, S. James. *Superstring Theory: The DNA of Reality.* The Great Courses. Chantilly, Va.: The Teaching Company, DVD, 2012.

Christ, Jesus. "The lamp of the body is my eye. If therefore your eye is good, your whole body will be full of light." Matthew 6:22, King James Bible.

Cayce, Edgar. *Edgar Cayce's Egypt: Psychic Revelations on the Most Fascinating Civilization Ever Known.* Virginia Beach, Va.: A.R.E. Press, 2004.

Herbert, Nick. *Faster Than Light: Superluminal Loopholes in Physics.* New York City, N.Y.: Penguin/New American Library, 1989.

Chandrasekharanand, Saraswati, S. Personal communication.

Jacobson, Edmund. *Progressive Relaxation.* Chicago, Ill.: University of Chicago Press, 1974.

Abbot, Edwin A. *Flatland: A Romance of Many Dimensions.* New York City, N.Y.: New American Library, 1984.

Schwaller de Lubicz, R. *Sacred Science: The King in Pharaonic Theocracy.* Rochester, Vt.: Inner Traditions, 1961.

Schwaller de Lubicz, R. P. *The Temple in Man.* Rochester, Vt.: Inner Traditions, 1998.

Bauval, Robert and Gilbert, Adrian. *The Orion Mystery: Unlocking the Secrets of the Pyramid.* New York City, N.Y.: Crown Publishing. Three Rivers Press, 1994.

Strieber, Whitney. *The Key.* New York, N.Y.: J.P. Tarcher, 2000.

Diop, Cheik A. *The African Origin of Civilization,* Brooklyn, N.Y.: Lawrence Hill Books, 1974.

Diop, Cheik A. *Civilization of Barbarism: An Authentic Anthropology.* Brooklyn, N.Y.:

Lawrence Hill Books, 1991.

Finch, Charles S. *Echoes of the Old Darkland: Themes from the African Eden.* Decatur, Ga.: Khenti Publishers, 1991.

Groth-Marnat, Gary. *Handbook of Psychological Assessment.* New York City, N.Y.: Wiley, 2003.

Kubie, Lawrence S. "The Ontogeny of Racial Prejudice." *Journal of Nervous and Mental Disease* 141 (3), (1965): 265-273.

Graff, Dale. *Tracks in the Psychic Wilderness: An Exploration of ESP, Remote Viewing,*
    Precognitive Dreaming and Synchronicity. Boston, Mass.: Element Books, 1998.

Monroe, Robert A. *Journeys Out the Body.* New York City, N.Y.: Doubleday and
    Company, 1977.

Goswani, Amit. *The Self-Aware Universe.* New York City, N.Y.: J.P.Tarcher, 1995.

Goswani, Amit. *Quantum Mechanics*. Dubuque, Ind.: William C. Brown, 1997.

Krauss, Lawrence M. "Cosmology: What is Dark Energy?" *Nature: International*
    Weekly Journal of Science 431, September 30, (2004):519-520.

Finch, Charles S. *The African Background to Medical Science.* London, UK.: Karnak
    House, 1990.

Krishna, Gopi. *Kundalini for the New Age: Selected Writings of Gopi Krishna.* Edited
    By Gene Kieffer. New York City, N.Y.: Bantam Books, 1988.

Laberge, Stephen. *Lucid Dreaming: The Power of Being Awake and Aware in*

Your
 Dreams. Jeremy P. Tarcher. Los Angeles, Calif.:1985.

Krishna, Gopi. *Kundalini, The Evolutionary Energy in Man.* New York City, N.Y.:
 Harper and Row, 1971.

Lynch, B. M. and Robbins, L.H. "Namoratunga: The First Archneoastronomical Evidence in Sub-Saharan Africa." *Science* 200, May 19, (1978): 766-768.

"Visible Human Project: Neural Line from Brain to Lower Spine."
 < http://www.nlm.nih.gov/research/visible> accessed 2010.

Gardiner, Philip. *Secrets of the Serpent: In Search of the Sacred Past.* Milton Keynes, UK.: Reality Press, 2006.

Gardiner, Philip. *Brotherhood of the Snake.* Seattle, Wash.: CreateSpace, 2007.

Eliade, Mircea. *Yoga: Immortality and Freedom.* Willard Trask (trans. from the French).
 Princeton, N.J.: Bollingen Series, Princeton University Press, 1958.

Hartsuker, Dolf. *Sadhus: India's Mystic Holy Men.* Rochester, Vt.: Inner Traditions, 1993.

Pinkham, Mark A. *The Return of the Serpents of Wisdom.* Kempton, Ill.: Adventures
 Unlimited Press, 1997.

Faro, S.H., Koenigsberg, R.A., Turtz, A.R. and Croul, S.E. "Melanocytoma of the
 Caverous Sinus: CT and MR Findings." *American Society of Neuroradiology,*
 June,(1996): 1087-1090.

Kung, B., Deschenes, G.R., Keane, W., Cunnane, M., Jacob-Ampuero, M.P., and Rosen, M. "Paranasal Sinus Melanoma Masquerading as Chronic

Sinusitis and Nasal Polyposis." *ENT-Ear, Nose and Throat Journal 86 (9)* September, (2007): 561-564.

Corti, A. "Recherches Surl'organe de L'ouic Mammiferes." *Premiere Partie* 2 *Wiss Zoologie* 3, (1851):109-169.

Wolf, D. "Melanin in the Inner Ear." *Archives in Otolaryngology* 14 (1931): 195-211.

Hilding, D.A. and Ginsberg, R.D. "Pigmentation of the Stria Vascularis." *Acta Otolaryngology, 84 (1977):24-37.*

LaFerriere, K.A., Arenberg, I.K. Hawkins, J.E. and Johnson, L.G. "Melanocytes of the
Vestibular Labyrinth and their Relationship to the Microvasculature." *Annals of Otology,* 83 (1974): 685-694.

Breathnach, A.S. "Extra-cutaneous Melanin." *Pigment Cell Research* 1 (1988): 234-237.

Adeloyem A. "Incidence of Normal Pineal Gland Calcification in Skull Roentgenograms of Black and White Americans." *American Journal of Roentgenology and Radiation
Therapy* 122 (1974): 481-484.

Daramola, G. F. and Olowu, A. O. "Physiological and radiological implications of low incidence of pineal calcification in Nigeria". Neuroendrocrinology, 9, (1972): 41-57.

Sannella, Lee. *The Kundalini Experience: Psychosis or Transcendence.* Lower Lake, Calif.: Integral Publishing, 1987.

Benton, Isaac. *Stalking the Wild Pendulum: On the Mechanics of Consciousness.*
New York City, N.Y.: Dutton Books, 1987.

Haich, Elizabeth. *Initiation.* New York City, N.Y.: Aurora Publishers, 2000.

Hoffman, Danielle R. *The Temples of Light: An Initiatory Journey into the*

Heart Teachings of the Egyptian Mystery Schools. Rochester, Vt.: Bear and Company, 2009.

Hall, Manly P. *The Secret Teachings of All Ages.* Radford, Va.: Wilder, 2007.

Schnapf, J. and Baylor, D.A. "How Photoreceptors Respond to Light." *Scientific American* 256 (4) April (1987): 40-47.

Hecht, S., Schlaer, S. and Pirenne, M.H. "Energy, Quanta and Vision." *Journal of the Optical Society of America* 38 (1942): 196-208.

Baylor, D.A., Lamb, T.D. and Yau, K.W. "Response of Retinal Rods to Single Photons." *Journal of Physiology,* Lond. 288 (1979): 613-634.

Griaule, Marcel and Dieterlen, Germaine. *The Pale Fox.* Chino Valley, Ariz.: Continuum Foundation, 1986.

De Chardin, Teihand. *The Phenomenon of Man.* New York City, N.Y.: Harper and Row, 1959.

Howell, Elizabeth F. *The Dissociative Mind.* Hillsdale, N.J.: Analytic Press, 2005.

Hill, H.G.M., Jones, K.P. and d'Hendecourt. "Diamonds in Carbon-Rich Proto-Planetary Nebulae." *Astronomy and Astrophysics* (1988): L41-L44.

Jenkins, John M. *Galactic Alignment: The Transformation of Consciousness According to Mayan, Egyptian, and Vedic Traditions.* Rochester, Vt.: Inner Traditions and Bear Company, 2002.

Jenny, Hans. *Cymatics: Structure and Dynamics of Waves and Vibrations.* New York City, N.Y.: Schocken Books, 1975.

Kaky, Michio. *Hyperspace: A Scientific Odyssey Through Parallel Universes,*

Time Warps, And the 10th Dimension. London, U.K.: Oxford University Press, 1994.

King, Richard D. *The African Origin of Biological Psychiatry.* Seymour-Smith, Germantown, Tenn.: 1990.

Kruzhevskii, B., M., Petrov, U., M., and Shestropalou, I., P. "On Radiation Conditions Forecasting in Interstellar Space." *Kosmicheskiye Issledovaniya (Space Research)* 31 (6) (1993): 89-103.

Laszlo, Ervin. *Science and the Akashic Field: An Integral Theory of Everything.* Rochester, Vt.: Inner Traditions, 2007.

Gyatso, Geshe K. *Clear Light of Bliss: Mahamudra in Vajrayana Buddhism.* London, U.K.: Wisdom Publications, 1982.

Cerami, Charles A. "The Dogon Ancestor" *Benjamin Banneker: Surveyor, Astronomer, Publisher, Patriot.* Appendix I. New York City, N.Y.: John Wiley and Sons, 2002.

Lockhart, Maureen. *The Subtle Energy Body: The Complete Guide.* Rochester, Vt.: Inner Traditions and Bear Company, 2010.

Knittle, E. and Jeanloz, R. "Earth's Core-Mantle Boundary: Results of Experiments At High Pressure and Temperatures." *Science* 251 March 22 (1991): 1438-1443.

Jeanloz, R. and Lay, T. "The Core-Mantle Boundary." *Scientific American* May (1993): 48-55.

Jeanloz, R. "The Nature of the Earth Core." *Annual Review of Earth and Planetary Sciences* 18 (1990): 357-386.

Thom, Alexander. "The Megalithic Unit of Length." *Journal of the Royal*

Statistical Society A 125 (1962): 243-251.

Mahler, Margaret S. *The Psychological Birth of the Human Infant.* New York City, N.Y.:
Basic Books, 1975.

Mookerjee, Ajit. *Kundalini: The Arousal of the Inner Energy.* Rochester, Vt.: Destiny
Books, 1982.

Miller, Iona. "Earth Works Series: Geomagnetism-Is the Earth Driving You Crazy?"
<http://www.sedonanomalies.com> accessed 2012

Murphy, C.J. et al. "Long-Range Photoinduced Electron Transfer Through a DNA Helix." *Science* 262 (5136) (1983): 1025-1029.

Pribram, Karl H. *Languages of the Brain: Experimental Paradoxes and Principles in
Neuropsychology.* New York City, N.Y.: Brandon House, 1971.

Pribram, Karl H. *Brain and Perception: Holonomy and Structure in Figural Processing.*
Hillsdale, N.J.: Lawrence Erlbraum Associates, 1991.

Cowan, James. *Mysteries of the Dream-Time: The Spiritual Life of Australian Aborigines.* Garden City, N.Y.: Avery Publishing Group, 1991.

Lawlor, Robert. *Voices of the First Day: Awakening in the Aboriginal Dreamtime.*
Rochester, Vt.: Inner Traditions, 1991.

Oyibo, Gabriel. *Highlights of the Grand Unified Theorem: Formulation of the Unified
Field Theory or the Theory of Everything.* New York City, N.Y.: Nova Science
Publishers, 2001.

Kazanis, D. "Dark Matter: The Physical Basis for Mysticism."
<http://www.active-stream.com/story/darkmatter.html> accessed 2006

De Buck, Adriaan. *The Egyptian Coffin Texts*.8 Volumes. The Oriental Institute.
Chicago, Ill.: 1935-1961.

Holzinger, B. and LaBerge, S.and Levitan, I. "Psychophysiological Correlates of
Lucid Dreaming." *Dreaming: Journal of the Association for the Study of Dreams* 16
(2) June (2006): 88-95.

Chia, Mantak. *The Healing Tao Journal.* Huntington, N.Y.: Healing Tao Books, 1989.

Leviton, R. "The Holographic Body." *East/West Journal* August (1988) 36-47.

Evans-Wentz, Walter Y. *The Tibtetan Book of the Dead (Bardo Thodol)* London, U.K.:
Oxford University Press, 1960.

Chandler, Wayne B. *Ancient Futur: The Teachings and Prophetic Wisdom of the Seven
Hermatic Laws of Ancient Egypt.* Atlanta, Ga.: Black Classic Press.

Kellicott, William E. *A Textbook of General Embryology.* New York City, N.Y.: Henry
Holt and Company, 1913.

Selman, G. G. "The Forces Producing Neural Closure in Amphibia." *Journal Embryological Exp. Morph.* Edinburgh, U.K.: (1958) 448-465.

Marsden, C. D. "Brain Pigment and its Relation to Brain Catecholamines." *The
Lancet.* September 4 (1965): 475-476.

Forrest, F. M. "Evolutionary Origin of Extrapyramidal Disorders in Drug-treated Mental Patients, its Significance, and the Role of Neuromelanin." *In the Phenothiazines and Structurally Related Drugs.* I.S. Forrest, CJ Carr, E.Usdin, editors. N.Y. Raven 255-268.

Saper C. B. and Petito, C. K. "Correspondence of Melanin-Pigmented Neurons in Human Brain with Ai-A14 Catecholamine Cell Gropus." *Brain* 105 (1982): 87-101.

Bogerts, B. "A Brainstem Atlas of Catecholaminergic Neurons in Man, Using Melanin as a Natural Marker." *Journal of Comparative Neurology* 197 (1981): 63-80.

Marsden, C. D. "Pigmentation in the Nucleus Substantia Nigra in Primates." *Journal Of Comparative Anatomy* V95 (1961): 162-256.

Sporns, Olaf. *Networks of the Brain.* Cambridge, Mass.: MTT Press, 2010.

Striedter, Georg, F. *Principles of Brain Evolution.* Sunderland, Mass.: Sinauer Associates, 2004.

Scherer H., J. "Melanin Pigmentation of the Substantia Nigra of Mammals." *Journal Of Comparative Anatomy* 71 (1939): 91-95.

Blois, Marsden S. *Recent Developments in the Physics of Chemistry of Melanin Pigmentation.* Elmsford, N.Y.: Pergamon Press, 1969.

Filators, J. and McGinnes, John. "Thermal and Electronic Contributions to Switching In Melanins." *Biopolymers* 15 (2309).

Barr, Fredrick E. *Melanin: The Organizing Molecule Medical Hypotheses* 11 (1983): 3-4.

Myers, Fredrick W. H. "The Subliminal Consciousness." *Chapter 1. General Characteristics of Subliminal Messages. Proceedings of the Society for Psychical Research* 7 (1891-2): 298-327.

Myers, Fredrick W. H. *Human Personality and its Survival of Bodily Death.* New York City, N.Y.: University Books, 1961 (originally published in 1903).

Cowan, David and Arnold, Chris. *Ley Lines and Earth Energies: A Ground-Breaking Exploration of the Earth Natural Energy and how it affects our Health.* Cottonwood, Ariz.: Adventures Unlimited Press, 2003.

Netter, Frank H. *The CIBA Collection of Medical Illustrations, Volume 1 Nervous System.* Summit, N.J.: CIBA Pharmaceutical Company, 1972.

Moore, Timothy O. *The Science of Melanin*. Redan, Ga.: Zamani Press, 2004.

King, Richard D. *African Origin of Biological Psychiatry.* Germantown, Tenn.: Seymour-Smith, 1990.

Winn, Philip. *Dictionary of Biological Psychology, Circumventricular Organs.* London, U.K.: Routledge, 2001.

McGinness, J. and Proctor, P. The Importance of the Fact that Melanin is Black."
Journal of Theoretical Biology 39 (1973): 677-688.

McGinness, J., Corry, P. and Proctor, P. "Amorphous Semiconductor Switching in Melanins." *Science* 183 (1974): 853-855.

Plato, *Timaeus.* Translated by Francis MacDonald Cornford. New York: Liberal Arts

Press, 1959.

Plato, *Plato Protagoras*. Translated by C.C.W. Taylor. Revised edition. London, U.K.:
Oxford University Press, 1990.

Ring, Kenneth. *Heading Toward Omega: In Search of the Meaning of the Near-Death
Experience*. New York City, N.Y.: Harper Perennial, 1985.

Ross, Colin A. *Dissociative Identity Disorder: Diagnosis, Clinical Features and Treatment of Multiple Personality*. New York City, N.Y.: John Wiley and Sons, 1997.

Targ, Russell and Puthoff, Harold E. *Mind-Reach: Scientists Look at Psychic Abilities*.
New York City, N.Y.: Delacorte, 1977.

Yukteswar, Swami S. *The Holy Science*. Los Angeles, Calif.: Self-Realization Fellowship
(original 1894), 1977.

Salaman, Clement, Van Oven, Dorine, Wharton, William D., Mahe, Jean-Pierre. *The Way of Hermes: New Translations of the Corpus Hermeticum and the Definitions of Hermes Trismegistus to Ascelepius*. Rochester, Vt.: Inner Traditions, 2004.

Ovason, David. *The Secret Architecture of Our Nation's Capital*. New York City, N.Y.:
Harper Collins, 2000.

Devereax, Paul. *Shamanism and the Mystery Lines: Ley Lines, Spirit Paths, Out-of-Body
Travel and Shape Shifting*. U.K.: Llewellyn Publications, 1993.

Cowan, David and Arnold, Chris. *Ley Lines and Earth Energies: A Groundbreaking
Exploration of the Earth's Natural Energy and how it affects our Health*. Kempton,

Ill.: Adventures Unlimited Press, 2003.

Mouritsen, H. and Ritz, T. "Magnetoreception and its use in Bird Navigation."
Current Opinion in Neurobiology 15 (4) August (2005).

Poynder, Michael. *Lost Science of the Stone Age: Sacred Energy and the I.Ching.* Somerset, U.K.: Green Magic Publishers, 2005.

Carlson, E. B. and Putnam, F. W. "An Update on the Dissociative Experiences Scale." *Dissociation.* Vol, V1 (1) March (1993): 16-27.

Ross, Colin A. *Dissociative Identity Disorder: Diagnosis, Clinical Features and
Treatment of Multiple Personality.* New York City, N.Y.: John Wiley and Sons, 1997.

Howell, Elizabeth F. *The Dissociative Mind.* Hillsdale, N.J.: Analytic Press, 2005.

Monastersky, R. "The Globe Inside Our Planet: Earth's Inner Core is Turning Out to be an Alien World." *Science News* 154 July 25 (1998): 58-60.

Hoffman, K. A. "Ancient Magnetic Reversals: Clues to the Geodynamo.' *Scientific American* May (1988): 77-83.

Sington, D. *Magnetic Storm: Earth's Invisible Shield.* NOVA. DVD Production.
WGBH Educational Foundation. Mass: Boston, 2003.

Cox, A. and Dalrymple, G. B. and Doell, R. R. "Reversals of the Earth's Magnetic Field." *Scientific American* 216 (1967): 44-54.

Barker, A. T. and Freeston, I. L. "Non-invasive Magnetic Stimulation of Human
Cortex." *The Lancet* 1 (8437) (1985): 1106-1107.

Rossi, P. and Rossi, S. "Transcranial Magnetic Stimulation: Diagnostics,

Therapeutic,
And Research Potential." *Neurology* 68 (7) (2007): 484-488.

Persinger, Michael. *ELF and VLF Electromagnetic Field Effects*. New York City, N.Y.:
Plenum, 1974.

Vusumazulu, Credo Mutwa. *The Song of the Stars: The Love of a Zulu Shaman.* Barrytown, N.Y.: Station Hill Openings, Barrytown Limited, 2000 (1995).

James, George G. M. *Stolen Legacy.* New York City, N.Y.: Philosophical Library,
United Brothers Communication Systems, 1954.

Svatmarama, Swami. *Hatha Yoga Pradipika (The Yoga of Light).* Trans. By Hans-Ulrich
Rieker. Trans. into English by Elsy Becherer. New York City, N.Y.: Herder and Herder Inc. and Dawn House Press, 1971.

Wickramasinghe, C. "The Astrobiological Case for our Cosmic Ancestry." *Int. Journal of*
Astrobiology 9 (2) (2010): 119-130.

West, John Anthony. *Serpent in the Sky: The High Wisdom of Ancient Egypt.* New York City, N.Y.: Harper and Row, 1979.

Zimmer, Heinrich. *Philosophies of India.* Princeton, N.J.: Princeton University Press, 1969.

Vygotsky, Lev S. S. *Thought and Language.* Cambridge, Mass.: MIT Press, 1986
(1934).

Khalsa, Siri Singh B.S.H.S. "Basic Spinal Energy Series." *Kundalini: Yoga/Sadhana*
Guidelines. Pomona, Calif.: Kundalini Research Institute of 3HO Foundation, 1978.

Rama, Sawmi., Ballentine, Rudoft., Hymes, Alan. *The Science of Breath: A Practical Guide.* Honesdale, Pa.: Himalayan International Institute, 1979.

Funderburk, James. *Science Studies Yoga.* Honesdale, Pa.: Himalayan International Institute, 1977.

Gepal, K.S., Anantharaman, V., Balachandar, S. and Nishith, S.D. "The Cardio-respirator Adjustments in Pranayama With and Withut Bandhas. *Indian Journal of Medical Science* 27 (9) (1973):

Rai, Ram, Kumar. *Shiva Svarodaya.* Translated by R.K. Rai. Chowkhamba Sanskrit Series Office. P.O. Box #8, Varanasi, India.:

Van Lysebeth, Andre. *Pranayama: The Yoga of Breathing.* London, England.: Unwin Paperbacks, 1983.

Singleton, Mark. "Yoga's Greater Truth." *Yoga Journal.* November (2010): 66-107.

Singleton, Mark. *Yoga Body: The Origins of Modern Posture Practice.* Oxford University Press, 2010.

Kuvalayananda, Swami. *Pranayama.* Philadelphia, Pa.: The Sky Foundation, 1978.

Lukoff, David. "Spiritual Emergency Network." <http://www.spiritualemergency.blogspot.com> accessed 2006.

Grof, Stanislav. *Spiritual Emergency: When Personal Transformation Becomes a A Crisis.* New York City, N.Y.: J.P. Tarcher, 1989.

Eriksson, P.S. and Perfilieva, E. and Bjork-Eriksson, T. and Alborn, A-M. and Nordborg, C., and Peterson, D.A. and Gage, F. "Neurogenesis in the Adult Hippocampus." *Nature Medicine* (1998): 1313-1317.

Kempermann, G. and Kuhn, H.G. and Gage, F.H. "Experience-induced Neurogenesis in the Senescent Dentate Gyrus." *Journal of Neuroscience* 18 (1998): 3206-3212.

Eckenhoff, M.F. and Rakic, P. "Nature and Fate of Proliferative Cells in the Hippocampal Dentate Gyrus During the Life Span of the Rhesus Monkey." *Journal of Neuroscienc e*8 (1988): 2729-2747.

Harrigan, Joan Shivarpita. *Kundalini Vidya: The Science of Spiritual Transformation.*
Knoxville, Tenn.: Patanjali Kundalini Yoga Care, 2002.

Narayanananda, Swami. *The Primal Power in Man or the Kundalini Shakti.* Gylling,
Denmark: N.U. Yoga Trust and Ashrama, 1979.

Scholem, Gershom. *Major Trends in Jewish Mysticism.* New York City, N.Y.: Schochen Books, 1974.

Chia, Mantak. *Awakening Healing Light of the Tao.* Aurora Press, 1983.

Huang, Di. *The Yellow Emperor's Classic of Medicine (The Neijing Suwen).* Boston, Mass.: Shambala Publications, 1995.

Hurtak, J.J. *The Keys of Enoch.* Los Gatos, Calif.: The Academic for Future Science, 1982.

Hecht, Laurence. "Advances in Developing the Moon Nuclear Model."
http://www.21stcenturysciencetech.com/articles/moon_nuc.html accessed 2012.

Hecht, Laurence. "The Geometric Basis for the Periodicity of the Elements." *21st Century*
18 May-June (1988):

Bhaskararaya. *Bhavanopanisad* (Translated by S. Mira). Madras, India: Ganesh and
Company, 1976.

Singh, Kirpal. *The Crown of Life: A Study in Yoga.* Delhi, India. :Ruhani Satsang Divine Science of the Soul. 1961.

Aurobindo, Ghosh, Sri. *The Life Divine.* Pondicherry, India: Sri Aurobindo Ashram Press, 1960.

Aurobindo, Ghosh, Sri. *The Synthesis of Yoga.* Pondicherry, India: Sri Aurobindo Press, 1955.

Mookerjee, Amit. *Kundalini: The Arousal of the Inner Energy.* Rochester, Vt.: Destiny Books, 1982.

Doreal (Translator) *The Emerald Tablets of Thoth.* Nashville, Tenn.: Source Books, 1925.

Motoyama, Hiroshi. *Theories of the Chakras: Bridge to Higher Consciousness.* Wheaton, Ill.: Theosophical Publishing House, 1981.

Iscariot, Judas. *The Gospel of Judas* (from Codex Tchacos), edited by Rodolphe Kasser, Marvin Meyer and Gregor Wurst. Washington D.C.: National Geographic, 2006.

Mack, John E. *Passport to the Cosmos: Human Transformation and Alien Encounters.* Guilford Surrey, U.K.: White Crow Books, 2010.

Mack, John E. *Abduction: Human Encounter with Aliens.* New York City, N.Y.: Scribner, 2007.

Franklin, Benjamin. "Letter to his niece Elizabeth Hubbart on the death of his brother." February 22 (1756), www.beliefnet.com accessed 2012.

Dyczkowski, Mark. *The Doctrine of Vibration: An Analysis of the Doctrines*

and
    Practices of Kashmir Shaivism. Albany, N.Y.: SUNY Press, 1987.

Lakshmanjoo, Swami. *Kashmir Shaivism: The Secret Supreme.* U.K.: Author
    House Books, 2003.

Shankarananda, Swami. *Consciousness is Everything: The Yoga of Kashmir Shaivism.*
    . : Shaktipat Press, 2003.

Ulansey, David. *The Origins of the Mithraic Mysteries.* London, U.K.: Oxford
    University Press, 1991.

Griaule, Marcel. *Conversations with Ogotemmeli.* London, U.K.: Oxford University
    Press, 1965.

Coleridge, Samuel Taylor. *Omniana of Samuel Taylor Coleridge: "The Universe".*
    Edited by T.Ashe. London, U.K.: George Bell and Sons, 1889.

Freud, Sigmund. "Freud's contributions to science", *Journal Harofe Haivri*, 1,1940, cited by Lionel Trilling in 'Freud and Literature' in *The Liberal Imagination*,1940.

Kafatos, Menas and Nadeau, Robert. *The Conscious Universe: Part and Whole in Modern Physical Theory.* NY, NY.: Springer-Verlag,1990.

Brief Autobiographical Statements

Edward Bruce Bynum, Ph.D., ABPP, is a licensed psychologist, Diplomate in clinical psychology and is currently Director of the Behavioral Medicine Clinic at the University of Massachusetts Health Services in Amherst Massachusetts. He is a Senior Fellow in the Society for Psychophysiology and Biofeedback (BICA). Dr. Bynum serves as a training and supervising psychologist in the American Psychological Association approved internship at the University where he trains other psychologists and clinical social workers during their internship year in hypnosis, psychosomatic medicine, computerized biofeedback, neurofeedback, and family therapy. He leads training seminars in dreams and cross-cultural psychology. Dr. Bynum has studied, trained and lectured in psychology in the United States, Africa and India.

Dr. Bynum is the author of numerous clinical articles in scientific journals, four texts in psychology and two in poetry. His most recent texts in psychology are **The African Unconscious: Roots of Ancient Mysticism And Modern Psychology** (Cosimo Books), **Families And The Interpretation of Dreams** (Paraview Special Books) and **DARK LIGHT CONSCIOUSNESS** (Inner Traditions & Bear Company). He is the producer of a ten part audio lecture series on science, psychology, spirituality and African psycho-historical and philosophical systems. He is a frequent speaker at national and international conferences and has appeared on radio, television and in documentaries. His research interests include depth psychology as it pertains to neuroscience, neuromelanin, consciousness research, as well as the analysis of dreams, family dynamics, the philosophy of science, ancient history, anthropology-archaeology and yoga. Dr. Bynum is the recepient of the **Abraham H. Maslow Award** of the

Division of Humanistic Psychology of the American Psychological Association for "outstanding and lasting contributions to the exploration of the fartherest reaches of human spirit".

He is married and the father of two sons. He lives in the Amherst Massachusetts area and is a practitioner of kundalini yoga. Dr. Bynum's website is www.obeliskfoundation.com

Richard D. King, MD, is a licensed psychiatrist and researcher in private practice in the Los Angeles County Department of Mental Health at the West Central Family Services Clinic. Dr. King is also psychiatric consultant to the Kedren Acute Psychiatric hospital working primarily with African-American and Hispanic populations. He presents at national conferences, is Executor of the Aquarian Spiritual Center and is a lecturer in the Black Gnostic Studies/Stolen Legacy series. Dr. King is the author of **The African Origin of Biological Psychiatry (Lushena Books)** and also **Melanin: A Key to Freedom (Lushena Books)**. Dr. King is the oldest of five children and the father of four who traces his family lineage from a line of Blacksmiths stretching back through North East Africa, Dahomey, Haiti, Jamaica, Puerto Rico and Louisiana to Los Angeles California.

Dr. King's current research focus is PTSD, schizophrenia, memory recall and stimulant and hallucinogenic substance abuse. Among his wider research interests is the exploration of the relationship of the dark matter of melanin/neuromelanin to dream states, trance dynamics and the architecture of sleep, including the neurophysiological correlates of disciplines developed to explore these states of expanded consciousness. Dr. King has a long-standing interest in ancient Kemetic Egyptian history and psychology. He can be reached at P.O. Box 56410, Los Angeles, CA 90056.

T. Owens Moore, Ph.D., is associate professor of psychology at Clark Atlanta University in Atlanta Georgia. He is a biomedical researcher and African-centered scholar/activist involved in a wide range of interdisciplinary studies. Professor Moore trained in physiological psychology and teaches both psychology and neuroscience. His undergraduate degree is from Lincoln University in Pennsylvania and he won both his M.S. and Ph.D. at Howard University. He is actively involved in the departments of Psychology, Biology and African-American Studies at Clark Atlanta University. Professor Moore is also a co-founder of the Neuroscience Institute at Morehouse School of Medicine and is a member of the National Science Foundation funded Center for Behavioral Neuroscience. Dr. Moore has federal funding to investigate the effects of hormones and neuropeptides on social behavior in rodents and explores learning paradigms that can be used to enhance education. Professor Moore is the author of two books in this area, **The Science of Melanin** (Zamani Press) and **Dark Matters, Dark Secrets** (Zamini Press).

Ann C. Brown, Ph.D., Anatomist/Hematologist, is a Professor and researcher in the Biology Department at Medgar Evers College/CUNY in Brooklyn, NY. Dr. Brown teaches Anatomy & Physiology, General Biology, Chordate Morphology, Chordate Development, and Human Health & Disease. She has written and published articles in several journals such as, Blood, In Vivo, etc. She mentors and advises students with career decisions in the health sciences and medicine.

Dr. Brown developed a course for nurses taught in the Biology Department entitled: "The Human Body in Health & Disease", and has recently published **A Laboratory Manual For The Human Body In Health And Disease** (Kendall/Hunt) which is used for the course. Dr. Brown has accompanied several students who participated in training programs that included lectures and laboratory workshops, sponsored by The Foundation for Advanced Education in the Sciences (FAES)d, Inc., at the National Institutes of Health (NIH). The programs included courses in MPSP "Special Topics in Biotechnology; DNA Microarrays and PCR; DNA Technology; Stem Cell Techniques and Research; and, Apoptosis and Cancer. Students who completed the training programs received three college credits.

Dr. Brown has presented papers at national science conferences (Quality Education for Minorities-QEM) in her areas of research interests. These areas include: neuromelanin in the brain and its disease implications; and also health and food choices and their impact on the health and well being of African Americans.Dr. Brown has been a professional health consultant for the last twenty years. She is a member of The New York Academy of Sciences, Metropolitan Association for College and University Biologists (MACUB), as well as a presenter to community groups on diseases that affect our populations.

Made in the USA
Las Vegas, NV
16 September 2022